GET IT OUT!

Eliminating the Cause of

Diverticulitis,
Kidney Stones,
Bladder Infections,
Cervical Dysplasia,
PMS,
Menopausal Discomfort,
Prostate Enlargement...
and More!

D1596746

GET IT OUT!

Eliminating the Cause of

Diverticulitis,
Kidney Stones,
Bladder Infections,
Cervical Dysplasia,
PMS,
Menopausal Discomfort,
Prostate Enlargement...
and More!

Sydney Ross Singer
Soma Grismaijer

ISCD
PRESS

Published by:

ISCD PRESS
P.O. Box 1880
Pahoa, Hawaii 96778
U.S.A.

ISCD PRESS is the publication branch of the Institute for the Study of Culturogenic Disease, a program of the Good Shepherd Foundation, Inc., a non-profit research and education foundation.

Library of Congress Catalogue Card Number (LCCN): 00-108649

ISBN: 1-930858-02-7

Other Books by Singer and Grismaijer:

Get It Up! Revealing the Simple Surprising Lifestyle that Causes Migraines, Alzheimer's, Stroke, Glaucoma, Sleep Apnea, Impotence…and More! (ISCD Press, HI 2000) ISBN 1-930858-00-0

Get It Off! Understanding the Cause of Breast Pain, Cysts, and Cancer, Illustrated with A Little Breast Play (ISCD Press, HI 2000) ISBN 1-930858-01-9

The Doctor Is Out! If you've been told you have high blood pressure, low thyroid, or diabetes, you may be a victim of one of the mist common medical scams of our time. (ISCD Press, HI 2001) ISBN 1-930858-04-3

Dressed To Kill: The Link Between Breast Cancer and Bras (Avery, NY 1995) ISBN 0-89529-664-0

Printed in Canada
10 9 8 7 6 5 4 3 2

Contents

Dear Reader

When someone politely asks about your health, there are probably some things you would not be willing to discuss. If you had arthritis or a sore back, no problem. And you would gladly discuss your headache or toothache. But when it comes to your recent flare-up of hemorrhoids, or your constipation, it's another story. You may be reluctant to tell others about having to get up a dozen times in the night to urinate, and that it takes forever to empty your bladder because your prostate is enlarged, and that urinating is now especially painful because you're still trying to recover from passing the biggest kidney stone your doctor has ever seen.

You would talk about your osteoporosis more easily than about your hot flashes. You may admit to burps, but not to farts.

There are certain taboo topics that we simply cannot discuss easily, if at all. Most people would not discuss their personal colon health or uterine cramping or prostate enlargement with a total stranger, except, perhaps, with their doctor. Many would not discuss it with a spouse or parent. And some cannot even think about it.

It is in the darkness of ignorance that health declines and disease flourishes. Whatever is taboo is shrouded in this darkness. We are culturally shamed by these taboos into regarding some of the most basic and essential aspects of life as unworthy of civilized, mature consideration. As a result, we suffer from diseases of apparently mysterious cause. Taboos blind us to the cause of these diseases.

Diverticulitis, kidney stones, menopausal discomforts, menstrual cramping, bladder infections, cervical dysplasia — these are all known to be lifestyle related, although the exact lifestyles responsible in each case is considered "unknown" by medical "experts", making one wonder why these people call themselves "experts". Theories abound, but none is definitive, and all require the purchase of some product, be it a pill, an herb, or a remedy; or of some service, be it surgery, massage, or colon cleansing. As a result of not knowing the cause, these diseases continue unabated, and generate a significant percentage of medical industry revenues.

Until the cause is known, the problems will recur, and may even progress into deeper forms of disease. We are going to show you that the cause is really very simple to understand, and to eliminate. It is embedded in certain cultural behaviors and attitudes about "nasty" topics. And it leads otherwise sensible people into doing extremely insensible things.

We will show you how the sensibilities of our society have desensitized us to our personal needs, and how this leads to various common diseases. We will explore this wasteland of disease, and explain what happens when our culture prevents us from experiencing our nature.

1

Taming the Beast

We are born into the world as naked, human animals - innocent, helpless, wild and free. Built within our little baby bodies is a natural wisdom that automatically guides us through life, healing us when we are ill, repairing us when we get injured, and progressively unfolding our very being as we grow and develop. It is a wisdom that also guides other creatures and beings who traverse this span of time we call life. It's all part of the Divine plan of nature. And it encompasses all life on Earth, connects us to the life supporting sun, and positions us within the cosmic framework of the heavens. It is the miracle of life.

For humans, however, there is another force within this play of life that further shapes and defines our path. It is powerful and inescapable, a force so compelling that people willingly kill and die for it. It takes over our minds and enslaves our souls. We come to identify more with it than with our own feelings, and learn to eagerly subordinate our sense of self to be part of it. And we come to firmly believe that we can't live without it, and we really cannot.

That force is our culture.

Our Culture

You cannot overstate the impact of culture on our lives. Culture takes the wild human and domesticates it. The culture clothes, feeds, punishes, rewards, manipulates, and, implicitly or explicitly, shapes people, creating a new form of human being, a person of a particular culture and at a certain time in the history of that culture. Depending on the tastes and norms of that culture, the people it produces will be different.

For example, how you place a baby down to sleep is medically known to alter head shape. A culture in which children are placed on their backs to sleep will produce rounder headed humans than in a culture in which children are placed down to sleep on their sides or stomachs. The ways this can alter brain function are now being studied. But it stands to reason that an expanding, growing brain may develop and operate differently in different shaped skulls. Structure and function go together. Put differently, when you change the structure of an organ, you change its function, as well.

Mothers are trained by their culture to treat their children a certain way, which is how the culture reproduces itself. Round-headed moms produce round-headed children. Of course, if you grew up in a culture of round-heads, you would never think about the fact that your head was round. Even though everyone you would speak with would also have a round head, you would never stop to think about it.

Oblivious to the Obvious

Actually, you never think about it *because* it is so obvious. We only think about subjects that catch our attention. It must stand out from the background of normal life. This means that we are typically oblivious to the obvious. And this creates a potential problem.

Continuing our example of head shape, let's assume that the brain works differently when it grows in a round head than in a more elliptical one. Let's make the assumption for this thought experiment that rounder skulls give more space and better circulation to certain centers of the brain, while at the same time providing less space and poorer circulation to others parts of the brain, relative to elliptical shaped heads. We would then expect that a round-headed culture would have different talents and strengths, as well as limitations and weaknesses, relative to an elliptical-headed culture. They might suffer from different brain diseases, engage in different activities, and have different attitudes. It would depend on how profound were the differences between the brains. And it would all stem, not from nature, but from nurture.

The Nurture of Nature

The simple act of placing a baby down to rest is one of a million nurturing acts that domesticates the human baby. Domestication, actually, begins before birth, inside the womb. The fetus samples the products of its mother's digestion. Is mom an anorexic, a fast food freak, a drug addict, an alcoholic, or a jalapeno pepper popper? It makes a difference to the fetus. Is that punk music playing or a Brahms lullaby? Is the pregnancy a blessing or a burden? It all affects the fetus. And it all reflects cultural attitudes, behaviors and values.

Then there is the delivery. While going through the process of exiting the womb, is the baby drugged as a side effect of mom being drugged by the doctor? Is the birth a natural delivery through the vagina, or a medical delivery through a Cesarean incision? When the baby is still within its first few days of life, will it be allowed to develop its immune system naturally, or will the baby's immune system be manipulated with vaccinations to create a culturally more acceptable form of development? And, if a boy, will the baby be altered anatomically by the surgical removal of the foreskin from one of the most sensitive parts of the infant's new body?

Human Domestication

The story of life has just begun, and so has the lifelong process of human domestication. We are beings defined by nature and born into a world defined by a culture. The wisdom of nature must conform to the demands of mortal mind. And the natural body designed to be well, healthy, and happy must be clothed in the cultural fashions of the times.

Nature is the rock from which a particular form of human is hewn. As we become sculpted into a particular type of cultural entity, nature is chiseled away from us. What was at first a wild, amorphous human becomes limited and defined in form and function. This is why people are born with so much more potential than they ever realize in their lifetimes. Nature endows us with great potential so that we might adapt to a wide variety of cultural realities that we may face as human beings.

While there seems to be a conflict between culture and nature, that only reflects the fact that nature places limits on what a culture can try to do. Ultimately, nature is in control. We can cheat nature a little and try to get away with it. But you always have to pay the price. When a culture promotes a behavior that is damaging to the natural requirements for health, the entire culture pays the price, and its people will get sick.

However, nature is merciful and allows us to get away with more than you would think possible. The human body has a remarkable ability to heal and a desire to live. We can insult our bodies with smoke, drugs, stress, poison, and clothing constriction, and yet we live. Some of us do. Others die as a result of trying to exceed the limits of nature. We humans love to test the limits. After all, you don't know where your limits are until you try to exceed them. And then it's too late. Or is it?

We Can All Heal

So long as people are alive and wanting to live, they have the ability to heal. That should be the credo of every person trying to recover from a disease and of every healing professional trying to help them. We were designed to heal. We were designed to work properly. The only problem is that our culture sometimes gets in the way.

We have mentioned some of the ways culture begins to domesticate the young human animal. As the process continues through life, all the natural functions of life become defined and controlled by the culture. How we eat, sleep, work and play are culturally prescribed. Some of these things are taught to us explicitly, through lessons and discussions. Others are taught implicitly, by following someone's example. Others are given to us without our knowing it, when we were infants. We are pressed into accepting these cultural attitudes and behaviors by parents, teachers, friends, and advertisers.

Education and Training

And the process works. You would call it brainwashing, if you didn't like the cultural content of what is impressed on the minds of those enculturated. Instead, we call it education and training.

What price do we pay for civilization? It is hard for those within that civilization to tell. Like the round-heads, we become oblivious to the obvious. But the reality that there is a problem is made clear by the presence of disease. We get diseased when we exceed the health limits of nature.

Culture-Caused Disease

As medical anthropologists, our task is to identify the cultural causes of disease. In 1995 we publicized our discovery that the primary cause of breast cancer is the compression and constriction of the breast tissue with bras. Our research findings, and the results of our 1991-1993 Bra and Breast Cancer Study, were published in our book, ***Dressed To Kill: The Link Between Breast Cancer and Bras*** (Avery, NY 1995). Just as some cultures bind feet for fashion, creating dysfunctional feet, women in modern western cultures bind breasts for fashion. The pressure from the bra on the breast tissue hampers proper circulation, and leads to fluid accumulation within the breast tissue. This causes cysts and pain, a condition called fibrocystic breast disease. Ultimately, low tissue oxygen coupled with reduced clearance of toxins from the congested breast tissue can lead to cancer. Once women forego the bra, their breasts experience improved health within weeks. Cysts go away, as does pain.

Breast Binding

Here, then, is a direct connection between culture and disease. Clothing is a cultural product. We are born naked. Clothing is an invention. Bras were invented to allow women to alter their breast shape. However, as you alter shape you alter function. Pressed breasts do not function as well as free, unrestrained breasts. Of course, the bra industry has sold the notion that the female body has evolved improperly, requiring 20th century lingerie for breast support. Girdles and corsets, which both have a medical history of damaging the body, were also rationalized by manufacturers, and by their hired medical "experts", as being necessary for maintaining body shape and for providing abdominal support. The bra, of course, is a breast corset. They are all just plain silly, and hazardous.

But bras are the cultural rage. And they are connected to more than breasts. The cultural issues surrounding breasts, sex, women, and body image blend with the images of fashion models and Barbie dolls, and creates a cultural image of a "woman" that looks the way fashion dictates, but just doesn't seem to work well. Something happens to their constricted breasts. They go bad.

We wrote, *Get It Off! Understanding the Cause of Breast Pain, Cysts, and Cancer, Illustrated with a Little Breast Play* (ISCD Press, HI 2001), to discuss the issues that have infected breast obsessed cultures with breast disease and cancer. Fortunately, the message is getting out to get the bra off, despite a lack of support by the medical community. Since medicine is the business that profits most from breast cancer and breast disease, deriving tens of billions of dollars annually from the treatment of these conditions, it

6

stands to reason that they would resist information about this primary source of their income. Medical leaders of the culture at the National Institutes of Health in Bethesda, Maryland, which is the nation's leading medical agency, as well as others at the American Cancer Society and the National Cancer Institute, are deliberately ignoring this obvious connection between breast disease and bras, and have insisted that this idea deserves no attention at all. (See *Get It Off!*) Meanwhile, open-minded, caring physicians who have been reading our books or have been talking with patients who have experienced for themselves the benefits of dressing bra-free, are realizing the truth of our claims and are prescribing bra abstention for breast disease treatment and prevention.

We made another discovery regarding a different culture-caused disease that has shaken the medical world and may prove to be a health panacea for people worldwide. This cultural problem relates to another obvious issue to which people have been oblivious. It has to do with sleep behavior. Our work started with our search for the cause of migraines. And our research took us into outer space.

Astronauts in space are known to develop migraines, glaucoma (increased eye pressure), and other manifestations of excessive head pressure. According to NASA scientists, fluid shifts to the head in the zero gravity environment of space. How do they research this zero gravity effect on Earth? They have subjects lie down flat.

Sleeping Too Flat

Gravity is a major force that affects the body. When the head is above the heart, which is the case when we are standing, gravity resists the flow of blood from the heart up to the brain, and assists the return of blood from the brain down to the heart. When we are lying down horizontally, the heart and head are on the same level, greatly reducing this gravity effect, causing fluid accumulation in the head and brain. This leads to increased pressure and congestion in facial and brain tissues, resulting in a condition called edema. Edema is a general term that refers to fluid accumulation in the tissues. (Swelling of the ankles at the end of the day is one form of edema.) This is an undesirable condition, since congested tissue soon starves of oxygen and nutrients and sits in its own waste. This can lead to tissue deterioration and dysfunction. Swelling of the brain causes internal brain compression, as well as compression of the sensitive brain tissue into the rigid skull. This condition, depending on its severity and duration, can result in anything from headaches or visual disturbances, to breathing difficulty, seizures, stroke, movement disorders such as Parkinson's disease, dementia disorders such as Alzheimer's disease, and more, including death.

While space scientists have known these facts about gravity and brain circulation, the implications for the health of people on Earth have been ignored. We reasoned that most people are sleeping too flat for too long each day, and that this causes excess pressure and fluid to accumulate in the head. When you wake up in the morning with stuffy sinuses, puffy eyes, and a congested feeling in the face, these are signs of this pressure and fluid accumulation. We also theorized that a migraine is the brain's way of eliminating congestion by forcing blood through the brain tissue to flush out stagnant fluid and replace it with fresh. In other words, a migraine is a brain flush. We had people with migraines test our theory, and found that they could eliminate migraines by elevating their heads 30-degrees while sleeping. We then realized that there are many diseases of allegedly unknown cause, also associated with brain congestion and/or pressure, which may also be related to head elevation and position while sleeping.

Get It Up!

Interestingly, head elevation while sleeping is a standard treatment for brain edema. It is often used to treat brain edema following brain surgery and trauma, in Reyes' syndrome, and following stroke. It involves the person sleeping at a 30-degree elevation, much as you would sleep in a recliner chair. This can ease breathing, too, and is used for stomach upset or gastritis, lung edema, and heart failure. However, head elevation has only been used to treat brain edema, not to prevent it. While space researchers knew that *lying* flat creates brain edema and pressure, and while doctors have used head elevation to treat brain pressure and edema, apparently none of the "experts" had ever thought that *sleeping* flat could create problems!

Our book describing this major disease prevention and treatment breakthrough is, ***Get It Up! Revealing the Simple Surprising Lifestyle that Causes Migraines, Alzheimer's, Stroke, Glaucoma, Sleep Apnea, Impotence, ...and More!*** (ISCD Press, HI 2001). The title suggests some of the many implications of this revolutionary new theory.

Amazingly, the cultural bias that assumes that sleeping flat is normal, and therefore is healthy, is what had blinded scientists to this simple realization. We contacted top scientists in the government and private foundations about this breakthrough that finally explains the mysteries of many brain conditions and diseases. They all agreed it made sense, and that it should have been realized long before now. But they all expressed doubt that anyone in the medical research world would be interested in following-up on our work. There's too much money being made treating these diseases, they explained. And the more we talked with the medical "experts" who do the treating and research, the more we realized that we were alone in our quest for prevention.

Medical Conflict of Interest

Here is another cultural cause of disease, as obvious as tight clothing and sleeping too flat. It's that the profit oriented medical industry has a monopoly and controls the health of modern, western nations.

It is a fact that in any capitalistic nation, profits come first. Profits are the purpose for business activity. Medicine is no exception. Even in non-profit hospitals or in cultures with socialized medicine, there are drug companies, high-tech medical machine manufacturers, surgical kit producers, and investors all making a living, or perhaps we should say a killing, on disease. When someone profits from the suffering of others, he becomes invested in that suffering continuing.

How does medicine get away with it? How can obvious lifestyle problems be ignored, especially after we have brought the issue to light? The answer is that they can't get away with it for long. In 20-30 years they'll have to give in. That's how long it typically takes for a medical breakthrough to become accepted by the conservative medical world. For example, it took 30 years for the American Cancer Society to acknowledge the possible relationship between tobacco smoking and cancer, and another 25 years for the National Cancer Institute to mention the issue.

Conservatism serves the medical leaders, since they like things just the way they are – with them in power. The only change those in power like is pocket change. It takes 20-30 years until these human impediments to progress retire or die. Truth can wait. But while it waits, uncountable numbers suffer because of the self-interest of a few.

There is one human factor that assists corrupted medical leaders in maintaining their control and power. It is that the causes of some health problems are so obvious that people are oblivious to them.

Cultural Traps

Most women ignore the red marks and indentations left by their bras that signal breast damage. Many a woman will admit, however, that the first thing she does when coming home, and is free from public gaze, is to remove her bra. But she would not have necessarily thought that this uncomfortable contraption was damaging her breasts.

Most people ignore the fact that they feel worse after sleeping, instead of feeling refreshed and invigorated, and that their heads feel pressurized when lying down. Many people will admit that they fall comfortably asleep in a recliner chair, but will insist that they must lie flat in bed to sleep. Questioning their sleep position and considering the health implications of spending one third of their lives horizontally in bed is something people are not trained, or even willing, to do — including doctors.

In fact, doctors are part of the culture, like everyone else. They fall for the same cultural traps that ensnare their patients. Most female doctors wear bras. And doctors sleep the same way as everyone else. They are equally oblivious to the obvious.

Obviously, what is obvious to one person may not be to another. This has become increasingly clear to us as we further our research into the cultural causes of disease. And now, we believe that we have uncovered the cultural cause of diverticulitis, bladder infections, kidney stones, yeast infections, cervical dysplasia and cancer, menopausal discomfort, prostate enlargement, and more. It is another cultural issue that binds us to certain attitudes and behaviors, while its obvious nature blinds us to the fact that it is causing so many diseases for so many people. It is a cultural issue that everyone deals with, but which no one will talk about. Shrouded in mystery and anxiety, it draws on subconscious impressions, and sometimes leaves us feeling embarrassed and alone. And it is something your doctor may never discuss with you, even after recognizing its truthfulness. It's something that plagues them, too. It is keeping millions of people frightened like children.

This makes sense, since it all started when we were still in diapers.

2

Diaper Daze

It is not long after the newborn comes into the life of its expectant family that certain new realities must be provided for. While the new parents peruse through parent magazine ads, wondering what outfit, crib, playpen, toys, and baby formula are best for baby Betty Lou, Betty Lou may be busy peeing on the bed. That's if the parents are lucky. She could have been pooping on the bed. That is why humans invented diapers.

Diapers are one of those cultural contraptions that we take for granted as essential. It is the first garment we wear. It hugs little bums, and stores all that nasty stuff that seems to collect in it every now and then, until we hear the baby cry or smell that it's time to change the diaper. When we think about diapers, we usually take the perspective of the parent or caretaker, operating as the infant's sanitation engineer. To such people, there is nothing as satisfying as a clean diaper on a clean baby bottom. At first, the stool of a baby is sweet smelling, since it is mostly milk product and the baby has not yet fully developed its intestinal bacterial population. Soon that all changes. The baby's digestion matures, and the stool more resembles an adult's in color, consistency, and odor.

Taboo Topics

Most adults in modern, western cultures, such as in the United States, have a hard time dealing with discussions of bodily

13

waste matter. While constipation and diarrhea are common maladies, as are bloating and flatulence, or farts, we typically do not discuss these problems in polite company. In fact, it is impolite to mention these issues in company, period. These are taboo topics. They are issues that the culture, for whatever reason, deems unsuitable for civilized conversation.

Civility is often the enemy of nature. When nature calls we are reminded that we are all animals, after all. Clothing, for example, is a civil façade stating our social rank and wealth. We use clothing to remind ourselves, and others, that we are civilized. When we are eliminating, however, it is our beast that must come out from underneath the clothing. We reveal our animal selves.

The goal of culture is to alter the natural. This means we lose our natural, animal selves when we become domesticated. A newborn that has just emerged from the womb through a vagina has no problem with the smell of stool. Stool is natural. Somehow, however, this changes, because most adults have a hard time dealing with excrement. Why do we become poop-phobic?

Poop-Phobia

It starts with the diaper. If we lived outdoors and with nature, as we imagine ancient Native Americans to have lived, we would allow our babies to run around naked as much as possible. Clothing has two major drawbacks that you can never get around. You need money to buy them, and you need to clean the clothes from time to time. This is very labor intensive, especially when the clothes are for a baby. We are accustomed to using disposable diapers, washing machines, and dryers. Third world people cannot afford much clothing, disposable or otherwise, and spend a great deal of time using a rock and the nearby stream, if they are lucky enough to have a stream, cleaning whatever clothing they do have. Consequently, many people in poor cultures tend to avoid diapers as too expensive in time and money.

When a baby has to eliminate and it is naked, you can see

in the baby's body language what he or she is about to do, and respond appropriately. When the baby is clothed, you must look for subtle facial gestures. A naked baby gives a clearer message to the caretaker that it's time to go to the potty. When you train a baby this way, it takes relatively little time to get the child conditioned to going to the potty to eliminate. Children like this probably have no issue with stool or urine, and people from these economically impoverished cultures usually have no problem with public toilets, outhouses, or baby poop.

Now, take the average western cultural citizen. We live in finely furnished, carpeted homes. We have expensive linens and rugs, and easily stained couch and loveseat upholstery. For us, a baby is a potential home hazard. The last thing we want is to see little Huey in the den making doo-doo on daddy's recliner, or trying to water the carpet to see if it grows like grass. For us, diapers are a must.

Of course, conscientious parents try to make sure that the diapers themselves don't damage the baby. Cloth diapers are sometimes fastened with large, sharp safety pins, which are not very safe. If you use disposable diapers, you must make sure that the elastic leg bands are not too tight, cutting off the leg circulation, and that the waist is the right size. It is impossible to get the correct sized waist, since the baby's stomach will change size with movement, amount of food, gas, and body position. What's too tight for one position is too loose for another. So you get elastic waistbands that stretch. But this also means that it is constantly pressing on the baby's belly and skin, which may cause skin irritation and indigestion.

Then there is the issue of diaper material. Whether it is cotton or polyester will make a difference to the baby, since cotton is much more comfortable. But economics may say which is used, regardless of what's good for the baby. And then you have to consider scented or unscented diapers, and which baby lotion or powder to use. Of course, these scents, fumes, and powders can irritate the baby's skin, nose and lungs, possibly leading to nasal and bronchial congestion and allergic reactions.

The Baby's View of Diapers

These are some of the considerations parents must make about their baby's diapers. Most parents probably don't think about these issues. They don't have to. The culture has major marketing strategies designed to lead parents to the right products to do the right things for their baby. At least, according to the culture's concept of "right".

What do diapers mean according to the baby? Imagine what it would be like having to wear a diaper and to be forced to defecate and urinate on yourself. Some adults, unfortunately, come to this condition as an outcome of disease, requiring an adult version of a diaper. However, infants are different. They do not have the experience and conceptual ability of an adult to reflect on their situation. They are new to the world. And all they know is diapers. This means that for an infant, it is normal and expected to urinate and defecate inside one's pants. If Mommy and Daddy think that that is a bad thing to do, reasons the infant, then what's their problem?

Eventually, of course, the parent will have a problem. Having trained the baby to get accustomed to eliminating in the diaper since birth, it becomes a difficult task to re-train the baby to eliminate elsewhere. When the parent wants the baby to go in the potty, rather than in the diaper, it requires that the baby be able to communicate its needs, in order to allow for enough time to get to the potty, take off the outer clothes and then the diaper, get positioned, and go. It takes a higher level of development for a baby to do this, waiting for the gratification of its natural urges and communicating that need to its caretaker, than it takes to simply walk over to the potty while naked and go. This means that the affluent child with diapers may take longer to potty train than a naked, "primitive" baby.

Potty Training

Two years of this is a long time to buy Pampers or hang diapers on the line. Little Huey and Betty Lou, now toddlers and getting around, are still defecating in their diapers, much to their mommas' and papas' dismay. Eventually, the kids catch on. It may be from the reflexive recoil you did when Huey had that particularly acrid diarrhea. It was in your face. The upper lips lifted with the nose. The universal sign of, "Yuck!" The baby saw that. Or Betty Lou may have heard your impatience when she dirtied her diaper just after you dressed her, making you now undress her, clean her, change her diaper, get her redressed, before you can get back to whatever you were doing. In both cases the message from the parents was clear. It is bad when you have to urinate and defecate.

Babies receiving negative feedback from their parents simply because they cannot give enough advance notice to get to the potty on time may begin to develop an attitude about elimination. Freud began the scientific inquiry into what he termed the "Anal Phase" of development. The reason why we go through this phase is not because we are human. It is because we are humans who are raised with diapers, forced to eliminate on ourselves to our discredit and shame. Elimination, one of the most fundamental processes of life, is made an issue because of a culture that must contain baby waste for later disposal. And it creates one of the first crises in the life of the child.

Of course, we are not advocating the indiscriminate elimination of waste by naked babies in any part of the home. We live in an indoor culture that makes infant nudity messy. This makes diapers a necessity. And what happens when it is cold and the baby needs clothing to keep warm? You can't have the baby soiling clothing by not having diapers on. Diapers seem unavoidable, at least in some situations. It's the best solution we have.

But what's the price?

Learning To Wait

When we train children to eliminate in the toilet, we must be able to get the child to do one basic new function – wait. Up until the time of toilet training, babies were content with their method of elimination, so long as it didn't take Mom or Dad or the day care worker too long to realize that the diaper needed changing. Anxious parents eager to see their new baby's digestion working properly are sometimes very pleased when the baby has a good, firm poop, a sign of health and vitality. So the baby goes from a stage of being rewarded for defecating in the diaper, to one of being scolded for not holding it in long enough to get to the toilet. Soon, the child learns more effectively how to hold it in. Eventually, the child should be as good at holding in waste and resisting the call of nature as any adult.

That's the price. We have learned to resist the call of nature. We must housebreak the human animal. We must teach people self-control. Unfortunately, the self that is controlled in this case is our natural self that manages how our bodies eliminate waste. We have learned to control urges from the bladder and colon, which is achieved by squeezing the tight, circular muscles, or sphincters, that surround and control the exits out of these organs. Sphincter control is what helps us hold in farts and poop. The pressure in the rectum and lower colon can become very high, and you can still hold it all in by contraction of your anal sphincter. And your bladder may feel as though it could burst, yet you can shut the bladder sphincter and hold it in until you are safely in a restroom. Potty training a baby, then, requires teaching the baby how to use their anal and bladder sphincter muscles, and to put up with the discomfort until a toilet is available.

Putting Nature on Hold

And here we see the hidden cost. When we train the child to hold it in when nature calls, we are training the child to put the call of nature on hold. This produces bodily discomfort and sometimes pain, which the child must learn to endure. When babies are forced to endure this discomfort, they usually cry and fuss. This is their natural side asking for the satisfaction of the biological need to eliminate. Over time, the baby must learn strategies for coping with this discomfort, since discomfort is the price we must all pay, adults as well as children, in being citizens of an indoor, crowded culture which requires that we eliminate bodily waste, not on demand, but at an appropriate time and place.

Ignoring Our Feelings

One of the best coping skills is to ignore one's feelings. The brain accomplishes this by lowering its sensitivity to the incoming nerve impulses from the bladder or colon that indicate that the organs are full and need emptying. In other words, we can learn to dampen our feelings and ignore them when we believe that there is nothing we can do about them. This is a good survival strategy for managing occasional discomforts without making everyone around you tired of hearing you complain. But should it be a daily strategy for managing one's elimination of waste?

In summary, humans in our culture are forced to hold in their waste and to ignore their feelings because of the cultural need to exercise bladder and bowel control. Bodily waste becomes a negative thing because of experiences with diapers and toilet training. The net result is a culture of adults who have a problem with defecation and urination, and chronically hold in their waste. What are the health consequences of holding it in?

The Colon

Let's examine the colon first. The colon, or large intestine, is the end part of a large digestive system that starts at the mouth and ends at the anus. The colon is a large hollow tube surrounded by muscular fibers that rhythmically contract to mix and propel the

19

processing food forward through the system. The large intestine starts at the lower right side of the abdomen where it meets the small intestines and the appendix, which is a small dead-ended sac. The colon then ascends the right side of the belly up to the liver at the lower ribs, where it makes a left turn to cross the belly near the stomach. When it reaches the left side of the belly, near the spleen, it starts down again, then makes an "S" curve to the center of the pelvis, and finally shoots straight down as it becomes the muscular rectum, which stores stool for elimination. The anal sphincter keeps the rectum closed to the outside.

When the rectum gets distended with stool, the expansion of the wall of the intestine sets off nerve signals that start contraction. Since the large intestine is essentially a hollow tube, this contraction, which comes in directional waves pulsing towards the anus, shortens the diameter of the tube, and squeezes the contents forward. If the stool has bulk and is not too dry, it moves well through the rectum, out the anus, and into the toilet bowl. If the stool is dry and has difficulty moving, you are constipated. This is uncomfortable since the rectal pressure continues unabated, and pressure mounts in the colon.

Diverticulitis

There is a very common disease of the colon that plagues western cultures but spares less affluent, more "primitive" cultures. It is called diverticulitis. This condition is long-term, or chronic, and gets worse as you age, suggesting that it is a lifestyle condition.

Why are chronic conditions most likely lifestyle caused? Nature has no investment in suffering. When an animal gets injured or ill, it either recovers or dies. Predators usually kill the disabled and suffering. So long as the cause of the injury or illness is removed, the body knows that it must heal quickly in order to survive. This means that acute, or sudden onset, problems are what the body is ready to manage. When the cause is not eliminated, an acute problem will recur, over and over again. If the cause is a daily activity, the afflicted individual will never recover from the acute problem, and it becomes chronic. They continually suffer.

This unnatural state only continues for two reasons. The first is that the lifestyle cause of the problem lingers and continues to insult the body. The second reason is that the culture protects the suffering from predators. This keeps the suffering alive, but not well.

Diverticulitis is a chronic disease. This means that it is caused by a continual problem. Could holding it in cause this problem?

First, let's explain what this disease involves. The wall of the colon has areas of varying degrees of thickness and muscularity. If you were to stretch the colon wall you would find areas of weakness, particularly where blood vessels traverse the colon wall. These areas are capable of expanding under pressure more than the rest of the intestinal wall, creating a balloon-like pocket in the wall of the colon. These pockets are called diverticula. You don't want these pockets in the wall of the colon because digestive matter can get inside them and remain packed in there, festering and irritating the pocket lining. This can lead to inflammation and infection, as well as bleeding, and the condition is then called diverticulitis, which means an inflammation of the diverticula. This painful condition is dangerous since it can lead to a hole in the colon wall. Leakage of fecal matter into the abdominal cavity can cause peritonitis, or an infection of the abdominal cavity, and can lead to death.

A Medical Mystery?

Medicine claims that it does not know the cause of this common affliction, although it is known to be related to excessive pressure in the colon. Realizing that it has something to do with lifestyle, it was theorized that the fiber content of the diet might be a factor. At first, doctors thought we should eat less fiber. That didn't work. Then they concluded that we need more fiber. That didn't work, either. But having a high fiber diet has been known to increase the frequency of bowel movements and ease of stool passage, so a high fiber diet has been recommended, anyway.

What could be the mysterious cause of increased colon pressure that can lead to this protrusion of the colon wall? Perhaps there is an obstruction. One form of obstruction could be compacted stool from constipation. High fiber may ease this problem. Other obstructions could be from tumors or abscesses, but these are further outcomes of disease, not the primary cause of the disease.

Holding It In

Perhaps the greatest cause of obstruction is one that is never mentioned. It is the obstruction caused by an anal sphincter held tightly closed because there is no restroom nearby. You may be on the freeway with bumper-to-bumper traffic and have the sudden urge to evacuate your colon. The pressure will build as the rectum reflexively contracts. But a well-trained person will be able to withstand the pressure, even if a slight sweat does begin to moisten the brow.

When you hold it in you cause the colon to maintain the pressure that it normally uses to push the stool out the anus. Where is this pressure going to go? If the exit is blocked, the pressure will push the stool into the colon wall. If this happens long enough and with great enough force, the colon wall may expand and bulge out in weak areas, like a balloon, forming diverticula.

This may be why a high fiber diet has failed to prevent diverticulitis. The fiber may make it easier to defecate. But you must actually defecate. Having more fiber without more opportunity to eliminate may make you all dressed up with no place to go, so to speak. So high fiber diets may help relieve constipation, which should help reduce the incidence of diverticulosis and diverticulitis. But they make us defecate more frequently and with greater force, due to the greater bulk, and the need to hold it in may result in a higher incidence of these diseases as a result of fiber. This is why the incidence of diverticulitis is as high in vegetarians as it is in meat eaters. We all hold it in, regardless of diet.

Flatulence

This is only part of the story, however. Besides stool, there is another product that we hold in that causes trouble. It is an essential part of the digestive process, but we have come to regard it as repulsive and disdainful. Of course, we are referring to flatulence.

Gas is a normal product of fermentation that occurs in our intestines. Food is propelled through the digestive tract by the aid of gas, in addition to intestinal wall contractions. A certain amount of gas is normal, as are farts. However, we just can't pass wind while at the boss's house for dinner, or while making a sales presentation, or while out on a date for the first time. Whether they are musical or silently odiferous, farting in public is almost as taboo as defecating in public. It reminds us that we are animals, after all. It is also probably a major reason why dogs are popular pets for the home. It gives everyone someone else to blame for the farts. Fortunately, dogs don't mind the blame, or the smell.

People who suffer from flatulence are those members of the culture who must maintain their image and status as upstanding members of the culture — managers, teachers, doctors, and clergymen. *The higher their status, the less acceptable the flatus.* They cannot fart in front of others without loss of face. Imagine the doctor coming into the examining room with you standing there half naked, ready for inspection. He takes out his tongue depressor, puts it in your mouth, and says, "Say, 'Ahhhh!'" And in the solemnity of the moment a squeaky little sound emanates from the doctor's bottom, as the small examination room begins to fill with that invisible, but clearly identifiable scent. Making matters worse, there is no dog in the room. This is every doctor's worst nightmare.

When you consider how many people hold in their farts it is no mystery that we have a culture plagued by diverticulitis. People in poor countries, who are used to the smells of body waste, typically fart on demand. They also have less colon disease. It's a trade-off. Either pass wind, or blow up. The choice is ours.

Now, it is not going to be popular to tell someone who suffers from excessive flatulence to simply let it rip. We must be sensitive to cultural pressures that we be good, well-mannered, toilet trained people. That is why medicine has ignored this simple conclusion, although flatulence has been identified as the major factor in diverticular disease. (See references.) Can you imagine a doctor telling someone with diverticulitis to fart more? The patient will get another doctor. On the other hand, it would be a boon to our culture if people could excuse their farts by saying, "Sorry! Doctor's orders!"

We can now see the depth of culture caused disease. Fart retention causes colon disease. But the solution is not as simple as farting. People cannot publicly fart without embarrassment. They cannot talk with their doctors about farting in public, since their doctors cannot fart in public, either. Resisting the need to defecate and fart is trained into us from infancy. The causes of diverticular disease, then, are our beliefs and attitudes about elimination, and our domestication that compels us to place the call of nature on hold.

Of course, defecation is only one form of elimination. We also need to eliminate urine. Now, what do you suppose happens when we hold that in?

3

Urine Trouble

Medicine has recognized four fundamental forms of elimination of waste from the body. These are defecation, urination, respiration, and perspiration.

Defecation removes unused foodstuffs from the digestive tract, as well as eliminates certain products from the body that have been processed and filtered from the blood by the liver. The liver is our toxin treatment organ, armed with enzymes to neutralize poisons and metabolic waste that travel to it through the bloodstream. It filters the blood, chemically alters these toxins, and stores some of them in the gallbladder, a pouch connected to the liver that also collects a digestive aid called bile. The contents of the gallbladder are emptied into the intestines during digestion, and the eliminated toxins can exit the body as part of the stool. In fact, the brown color of stool is due to certain substances produced by the liver in the breakdown of hemoglobin, the red protein within red blood cells that carries oxygen. Defecation, therefore, eliminates waste products created by the body, in addition to indigestible parts of our meals.

Bile and Toxins

Certain substances need to be eliminated from the body in stool, particularly fatty substances or those not easily eliminated in water. The bile in the gallbladder helps to stabilize these fatty waste products, since bile is an emulsifier. An emulsifier allows the better mixing of fat within the watery medium of the intestines. Bile serves the dual functions of aiding fat digestion in the intestines, by emulsifying dietary fat to afford greater enzymatic digestion, and of acting as a carrier of the fatty toxins that are being disposed of by the liver.

Respiration

The lungs are responsible for eliminating other substances, usually those that are volatile, or gaseous. Alcohol, for example, is eliminated in the breath, which is why drinkers smell like alcohol when they exhale. Bad breath is sometimes an indication that we are eliminating waste gasses through the lungs. Water-soluble toxins may also be excreted by the lungs, which carry them away from the body in the moisture of our breath.

Urination

Urination is the key method of eliminating toxins that can be dissolved in water. The kidneys are filters that selectively choose which substances need to be kept in the body and which need to be washed out, and they control the water and salt levels needed by the body. The kidneys are located towards the back, protected by the lower back ribs. They are nestled in dense fat pads that help absorb shocks to the area. The heart provides the pressure for the filtration of blood by the kidneys. Once the kidneys filter the blood and correct for the best urine concentration given current body conditions, the urine collects in collecting ducts and passively drains downward, by the force of gravity, to the bladder, which lies lower down in the pelvis. This assumes, of course, that the person is standing, or vertical. When lying horizontally, this gravity assistance is reduced, and filling of the bladder may be hampered.

The bladder is a distensible pouch that has two openings at the top, one for each kidney, that allow the urine in, and one opening at the bottom, controlled by a sphincter, that lets the urine out. Up to this point, men and women are pretty much the same. We'll get to the differences in a moment.

When the bladder is full, the distention of the bladder wall reflexively starts contractions, as is the case for the colon. When we resist the urge to urinate by keeping the sphincter closed, the pressure within the bladder builds. This leads to further distention of the bladder wall. Additionally, the pressure in the bladder can inhibit new urine from entering the bladder from the kidneys. This leads to increased pressure within the collecting tubes leading from the kidneys to the bladder. Ultimately, this translates into greater pressure within the kidneys themselves. Each kidney is contained within a tightly fitting capsule that maintains kidney size and integrity under normal conditions, and this capsule resists the added pressure in the kidneys caused by this back up of fluid from the bladder. This makes kidney pressure higher than normal, which leads to reduced filtration of the blood by the kidneys. Now the problem affects the rest of the body, since the kidneys are no longer doing their job well. Toxins cannot be eliminated, and water and electrolyte, or salt, levels cannot be adequately controlled. This can lead to heart disease, high blood pressure, and other problems associated with kidney failure.

The body, however, tries to do what it can to mitigate the problem. The bladder has the ability to concentrate urine, and it does this to reduce the pressure back-up we have just described. This is why urine becomes concentrated after we have been holding it in for a long time. Some of the water is absorbed through the bladder lining, leaving saltier urine behind.

Urine Retention and Kidney Stones

We can now see what can happen from urine retention. We make ourselves toxic by impairing renal, or kidney, function. And we end up with concentrated urine. What can that cause? The answer is simple. What can happen when you concentrate a salt solution, which is all that urine really is? The answer is that it can create crystals. In medicine, these are called stones.

Doctors say that they do not know the cause of kidney stones, while researchers study each stone's chemical constitution in a vain attempt to understand why it formed. The typical prevention advice given to stone sufferers is to drink more water. It is known that water can dissolve stones, just as it is known that concentrating a salt solution can form them. It's basic chemistry. However, drinking more is the solution only if drinking too little was the cause. For some people, this may be the case. Dehydration can lead to concentrated urine and stones. But the greater issue, the cultural problem, has been overlooked. It is not that people need to drink more; they need to urinate more!

Holding in urine, then, can cause kidney stones and bladder stones, as well as lead to heart, circulatory, and metabolic disorders due to reduced kidney function. But there is more it can do, which relates to the distention of the bladder.

Bladder Infections

When concentrated urine is chronically filling the bladder, the lining of the pressurized bladder can become irritated. This may lead to increased susceptibility to infections. Bladder infections, then, may result from urine retention.

Prostate Enlargement

Additionally, when a man is vertical, as when standing or sitting, the bladder is positioned directly above the prostate gland. The outflow of urine must pass from the bladder through the prostate gland, before it enters the penis for final exit. The prostate gland produces fluid that mixes with sperm during ejaculation. Even though the prostate is a sex gland, it must be traversed by urine every time a man urinates.

When you look at the anatomy of the lower pelvis you will see that the bladder lies above the prostate and the pelvic floor lies directly underneath it. This means that the bladder and pelvic floor make a prostate sandwich. As the bladder expands, the prostate gets smashed down onto the pelvic floor, compressing the prostate. To maintain its integrity, the prostate enlarges its mass, better resisting the weight of the bladder. As the prostate enlarges, the urethra, which is the urine passageway through the prostate and into the penis, gets constricted, preventing complete bladder emptying and requiring frequent urination. Enlarged prostates plague many men in their older years, a sign that it is the outcome of years of mismanagement of their urinary needs.

In summary, holding in urine can cause it to concentrate, producing bladder and kidney stones. And it causes distention of the bladder, producing bladder infections and causing pressure on the prostate, leading to prostate enlargement. Not surprisingly, these problems are greater in affluent cultures, where elimination is taboo. This means that our culture is giving us kidney, bladder and prostate problems. Doesn't that piss you off?

4

No Sweat

We have discussed the need for elimination by defecation, urination, and respiration. It is difficult to hold one's breath, so breath retention is not nearly the problem as urine and fecal retention. We have shown that a cultural problem has been created around elimination through the use of diapers and the need to domesticate and housebreak the human animal. By fostering a behavior of waste retention, the culture has caused people to develop diverticulosis and diverticulitis, bladder infections, kidney and bladder stones, and prostate enlargement.

Perspiration

So far we have not discussed the final major form of elimination – sweating. Unlike defecation and urination, sweating is not connected to early life diaper experiences. However, it is clear that modern civilization is not happy with sweating. Men can sweat, and typically do so. For women, however, sweating is an unappealing activity. Part of the problem is that sweat can ruin your make-up and hairdo. The last thing a woman needs is to start sweating on a hot afternoon at work, and have her mascara trace lines down her face.

Then, there is the smell. Sweat, which is similar to dilute urine, does not smell by itself. However, bacteria and fungi live on our skin, and in nasty places like the armpits and groin, and these like to eat our sweat, producing aromatic waste products that we call body odor, or B.O.. You can try to cover it up with perfume, but you risk smelling like a bull in a bordello.

Of course, there are also those unsightly stains and wet spots that cover the armpits of shirts and blouses. Nothing is more embarrassing than raising your arms to reveal a yellow armpit stain on your shirt, except, perhaps, farting at the same time. In short, sweat is an embarrassment, causing smudges, smells, and stains.

It is hard to hold in sweat. In fact, it is impossible, except perhaps for some well-trained yogi, since sweating is an automatic response. That is why some people use antiperspirants. These substances inhibit the sweating process. Others use deodorants, which are like bathroom spray for armpits. Deodorant use indicates one's discomfort with natural body odors, another cultural attitude that alienates us from our animal selves, although body deodorants may make it easier to breathe in the subway during rush hour. Deodorants are less hazardous than antiperspirants, since they still allow you to sweat. Antiperspirants keep you from properly eliminating the substances that need to be sweated out.

Sweat and Urine

Because sweat is similar in constitution to urine, we can compensate for reduced sweating by increasing urinary output. This makes the kidneys work harder. If the kidneys are already burdened, this extra work may be too much for the kidneys to manage. So, for example, a woman who uses antiperspirant and at the same time holds in her urine and refuses to defecate while away from home is a candidate for problems. She may develop toxemia, as waste products accumulate in her blood and tissues. Since respiration is also a form of elimination, some of these toxins may exit in the exhaled water and air that come from the lungs. This can give bad breath, which, if she is aware of it, she will most likely try to cover up with mouthwash or perfumed candy.

Retaining Waste

It should be no surprise to the reader that it is important to answer nature's call. Retaining waste cannot be good for you. Yet, little is ever mentioned about this problem, due to the taboos that enshroud it. As a test of our understanding of the problem, we reasoned that there would be more colon, bladder, and kidney problems among certain occupations than others, relating to the availability of restrooms. Jobs that make elimination difficult should have a higher incidence of these problems than jobs that make it easy to relieve oneself. To test this conclusion, we contacted the bus drivers' union in Victoria, British Columbia. Since bus drivers are on a schedule, they do not have the luxury of a nearby toilet, as office workers do. What we discovered was that a lack of bathrooms has been torturing these drivers. Some drivers are on routes with no restroom, making the drivers hold it in for their entire 7 1/2-hour shifts. If desperate, the driver must stop the bus full of people and quickly hop into a restaurant restroom, leaving the passengers on the bus waiting impatiently as they hope the driver simply has to urinate. The drivers sometimes get complaints from unsympathetic riders who are made late because of the unscheduled pit stop. Since the restaurant managers may not like drivers using their restaurant as a restroom stop, the drivers frequently feel compelled to purchase a drink, such as coffee. Coffee is a diuretic, meaning that it makes you need to urinate more, making the problem all the worse. As a result, many drivers opt to stay dehydrated, rather than to suffer from a bloated bladder.

Dehydration leads to constipation, which is another problem for these drivers. Urination is difficult enough to manage. Defecation is out of the question. And diarrhea is a nightmare. As a result of this pressure, bus drivers sweat profusely. The local union leader told me that the drivers' seats are usually soaked with sweat after their shifts. Antiperspirants would be useless. The entire shirt and pants are sometimes soaked with sweat. And, yes, bus drivers do have a high incidence of colon disease, including hemorrhoids, kidney stones, bladder problems, as well as blood vessel disease and heart disease.

Fortunately for these drivers, their union used the information we provided them about the hazards of holding in waste. At the time, the union was in negotiations with the city over a new contract. They had wanted more restroom facilities for drivers, but had been ignored in previous years' negotiations. We sent a letter to the local newspaper, the *Times Colonist*, and the issue became public. The union then successfully negotiated receiving about $20,000 a year to build new restroom facilities for its drivers.

Nature Over Culture

This story shows the triumph of nature over culture. There must be room in our culture for elimination, even though our schedules and the availability of bathrooms can limit the opportunities. We can only deny our needs for so long until it makes us sick.

We have now discussed the four major forms of elimination considered in medicine. There are other forms of elimination that are important, but are not discussed as forms of elimination. Spitting is a form of elimination, as is tearing of the eyes. We eliminate through the loss of dead skin and hair. Abscesses and pustules are also a form of elimination. In fact, every biological process that takes fluid or cells away from the body can be a vehicle for eliminating waste products.

Of all these additional forms of elimination, the most important one is a form of elimination that only women can do. It's called menstruation. And it can sometimes get women into a bloody mess.

5

The Ragtime Blues

Not long after a child is fully capable of retaining waste, it is time for puberty. For boys, this means nocturnal emissions, stronger smelling sweat, and facial hair. For girls, this means menstrual periods.

The Estrogen Cycle

Menstruation is actually a monthly cleansing. Throughout the month, the female body undergoes a rise and fall of estrogen, which is a female sex hormone produced primarily by the ovaries. Men have estrogen, too, but not in the same proportions as women. And men do not go through a monthly estrogen cycle as women do. In a series of hormonal maneuvers involving the hypothalamus and pituitary gland of the brain along with the ovaries, estrogen levels rise, and, if there is no pregnancy, they then fall sharply a few days before the menstrual period, which is when the woman bleeds. The bleeding is normal and comes from the lining of the uterus. If a fetus is growing in the uterus, the hormone levels adjust to the pregnancy, and the uterine lining, called the endometrium, stays intact. Otherwise, if not sustained by the hormones of pregnancy, the endometrium deteriorates and is excreted through the vagina and out the body.

Estrogen and Pre-Menstrual Syndrome, or PMS

As a result of elevated estrogen, the body retains water. Tissues swell with this retained water, which can create edema in various parts of the body, leading to discomfort, bloating, irritability, and general malaise. This is the origin of PMS, or Pre-Menstrual Syndrome. Soon, however, the estrogen level drops and the water is released from the tissues. The released water carries with it waste products from the tissues, effectively cleansing the body. These products are excreted in the urine, feces, sweat, and respiration, as well as in the menstrual flow.

The endometrium receives a large supply of blood prior to the period, allowing toxins in the blood to become absorbed by the endometrial tissue. As the tissue breaks down and leaves the body, it takes these toxins with it. Menstruation, then, is a monthly cleansing.

Needless to say, a culture with an elimination problem is not going to be comfortable with menstruation, either. How is a woman to manage this monthly bleeding?

Managing the Blood

Some cultures consider menstruating women "unclean", and insist that they stay in a special building or area among other menstruating women. They are relieved of normal duties, and must be avoided by others within their community. In modern western cultures, women can live normal lives while menstruating, so long as they keep their bleeding under control. Some women place a pad of cloth or other absorbent material between the legs to catch the drips of blood. But this can make movement limited, as the pad responds to the force of gravity. Another alternative is to place the pad inside of the vagina, at which time the pad is called a tampon. This is the most common method young women use to control menstrual flow. Tampons afford freer movement, since the tampon cannot drop out of the vagina. And the vagina has few nerve endings, making it minimally sensitive to the inserted object.

Tampons and Cervical Dysplasia

Soma's daughter, Camela, once came to us with a serious look on her 18-year-old face. She had been repeatedly experiencing a mucus discharge from her vagina for about a week following her periods, and it concerned her. Before telling us about the problem, she had secretly gone to a woman's health center, asking what could be causing the discharge. She was given a Pap smear to test the health of her cervix. The cervix is the muscular opening of the uterus separating the uterus from the vagina. In a Pap smear, an object, such as a wooden stick, is inserted into the vagina to rub cells off of the cervix. The cells are then spread onto a microscope slide. A pathologist then looks for abnormal cells.

In Camela's case, the report from the pathologist indicated that she had "atypical cells of unknown significance". She was told to return in a few months for another smear of her cervix. Nothing was mentioned about the mucus discharge. No cause of the problem was considered. She was just being watched to determine whether the condition would get any worse. Three anxious months of the same problem passed. Then Camela returned to the clinic. The results of the following test were alarming. "Cervical dysplasia" was the diagnosis, with a recommendation that she consider getting a biopsy of the cervix to check if it was developing cancer.

It was at that point that Camela came to us. What do you say to someone with a vaginal and cervical problem? We asked what she was doing to her cervix and vagina that was unnatural. When an organ has a problem, the cause is usually in something we have done to that organ. "Do you use tampons," we asked. She admitted that she regularly did, for each day of her menstrual flow. The answer was then clear.

Tampons and Irritation

A tampon is a wad of absorbent material that sticks to soft, moist tissue. If you were to place a tampon in the cheek of your mouth for several days, your cheek would be raw and irritated. The vaginal lining is similar to the lining inside the cheek, and will also become irritated by the tampon. In order to soothe the irritation, the mucus glands in the vaginal skin secrete more mucus, which is why Camela had a heavy mucus discharge following each period. Her vagina was trying to heal from the tampon irritation. In addition, the tampon pushes against the cervix, rubbing it with each movement of the woman's legs and pelvis. Constant irritation to the surface of the cervix will cause a similar reaction as constant irritation of the skin on the hand. It will create more skin to compensate, forming on the cervix the equivalent of a callous. This is the origin of the abnormal cells. Dysplasia simply means abnormal cell growth. A callous is a form of dysplasia.

While the tampon is irritating the area, it is soaked with the menstrual effluent. This means that toxins are being stored in the irritated vagina. Some toxins, of course, will be reabsorbed through the vaginal wall, particularly since the protective mucus lining may already have been stripped in places by the tampon. Tampons are known to cause micro-ulceration of the vaginal lining. This means that the tampon creates areas of raw vaginal tissue.

Cervical dysplasia can be a sign of cancer developing, which is what the doctors are looking for. But it is most likely a sign of cervical irritation from tampons. We advised Camela to get rid of the tampons and never use them again. Her mucus discharges stopped. Within months her cervix was healthy.

Tampons and Toxic Shock, Vaginitis, & Vaginal Ulcers

Tampons can cause toxic shock syndrome, vaginitis, and vaginal ulcers. (See references.) They are considered a type of medical device because of their potential hazards. When Camela received instructions from the clinic on what to do for a cervical biopsy, it explained that tampons should not be used for several weeks following the incision into the cervix. The reason? It was because the tampon could irritate the cervix. What about tampons irritating the cervix *before* the biopsy? Nothing was mentioned.

We have since met numerous young women with the same set of symptoms – mucus discharge after their period, and a diagnosis of cervical dysplasia. All of these women used tampons. Having not eliminated the cause, however, some of these young women went on to get biopsies. During a biopsy a chunk of cervix is cut away for a pathologist to examine microscopically. This is minor surgery that involves the possible risks of excessive bleeding, cervical scarring, and infection, and is performed merely for diagnostic purposes. The excuse made for subjecting women to this is that the dysplasia may develop into cancer.

Tampons can clearly cause the dysplasia. Could tampon usage lead to cervical cancer?

Cervical Cancer and Tampons

The manufacturers of tampons sometimes use fragrances or deodorants in their products to make the vagina smell springtime fresh, and to distract the mind from the culturally offensive act of managing menstrual blood. Some women have adverse skin reactions to these perfumes, which can irritate the mucus membranes and be absorbed through those membranes to enter the deeper tissue. There is also the process of bleaching the tampon material and processing it, which requires chemicals, some of which remain in the tampon material and may leach out, damaging the tissue.

Tampons may create an environment ripe for vaginal infections, including viral and yeast infections, due to the irritation of the mucus membrane in the vagina that makes the tissue more susceptible to offending organisms. And the tampons may be damaging the cervix and vagina by mechanical irritation, making it more susceptible to viruses and chemical irritants, especially chemicals leaching out of the tampons themselves. These chemicals may prove to be cancer causing.

Incidentally, some women are incorrectly diagnosed as having cervical cancer. A diagnosis of cervical dysplasia is easily considered a pre-cancerous state, so doctors can call it an early stage of cancer. But this is a sales ploy. When non-cancerous tissue is considered pre-cancerous, it makes it seem as though the cancer has already started, when it really hasn't. This is also a problem in the breast cancer field. The concept of "early detection" allows every lump and slight abnormality to be considered a potential cancer. Women, therefore, may be falsely diagnosed with cancer because of a cancer hungry medical industry.

Many of these results of tampon usage may make doctors jump to the conclusion that cancer is imminent, and that surgery and medication, along with regular check-ups and billable office visits, are necessary. Once patients are told that they are pre-cancerous, they become faithful customers. And unless these women stop wearing tampons, their doctor's expectations may become their personal realities.

Uterine Cancer

Chemicals released from the tampons can also enter the uterus, since the uterus is on the other side of the cervix from the vagina. However, uterine cancer is a major cancer for women, much more prevalent than cervical cancer, which suggests that it is caused by something other than tampons. Most uterine cancers are of the endometrium and occur after a woman stops menstruating and has entered menopause. As an eliminatory organ, the endometrium gets exposed to numerous toxins, some of which are cancer causing, or carcinogenic. We get exposed to carcinogens in our petrochemically produced food, in our polluted air and water, and in medications. These cancer-causing chemicals course throughout our bodies, entering all our tissues. While a woman is menstruating, she monthly cleanses her tissues of these toxins to some degree, bringing them to the uterus for elimination. But the repeated exposure of the uterus to these toxins may ultimately damage the uterus itself. And once menstruation ends, when a woman reaches menopause, the uterus can no longer clean itself by eliminating the endometrium. Of course, this is not good for the uterus, and may explain why it goes on to develop cancer.

Tight Clothing

There are other causes of uterine cancer besides the model we have just presented of toxin elimination. From our breast cancer work, we are exceedingly aware of the hazards of tight clothing, which restricts the circulation and hampers the immune clean-up of the tissues. Constricted tissue becomes low in oxygen, reducing all cellular functions, including those that protect the tissue from cancer and infections. Low oxygenated tissue also produces "free radicals" and other chemical products that damage cells and can actually cause cancers.

Some cases of uterine cancer may be caused by constriction of the pelvis by girdles, pantyhose, corsets, or even tight jeans or underwear. The pressure of the garment is transmitted through the body to the deeper organs, and may lead to reduced blood and lymphatic circulation in the uterus. The cells of the uterus, like all cells of the body, are bathed in a fluid medium, called lymph. The lymphatic fluid in the uterus must return to the bloodstream by traveling through lymphatic vessels and against gravity to return to the heart. Compression of the waist by constrictive, elasticized clothing may to some degree cut off this return of fluid from the uterus, leading to fluid accumulation within the uterine tissue. This may cause uterine cysts and pain. Cysts that linger from chronic constriction of the organ can become thickened with scar tissue, leading to fibroids. Ultimately, toxins accumulate in the organ from a lack of proper lymphatic cleansing of the tissue, which may lead to further deterioration and, ultimately, to cancer. The uterus, then, may suffer from tight clothing around the waist in the same way as the breasts suffer from bras. Constriction from clothing causes fluid back-up in the organ, leading to disease.

Interestingly, the parts of the body with the highest incidence of cancer are the lungs, breasts, colon, uterus (prostate for men), and urinary tract. If you notice, all of these are eliminatory organs, except, perhaps, for the breasts and prostate. The eliminatory organs must manage our poisons and waste. It is no surprise that they suffer most from cancer.

As for the breasts, they are known to produce toxic milk if the mother had been exposed to toxins, as though the breasts were eliminatory organs, too. This makes no sense in the natural scheme of things, since nature would not want mothers to eliminate into their infants' mouths. On the other hand, the toxins that we are exposed to these days that can be found in milk, such as pesticide and herbicide residues like DDT, are unnatural, and the body may never have anticipated their presence in the creation of toxic milk. In any event, this illustrates another point about the body. Any organ that can secrete a substance to the outside of the body can excrete, as well.

Secretions and Excretions

Cells produce secretions. When these secretions are considered by us to be waste products, we call these secretions "excretions". Excretions are simply unwanted secretions. If we lived in a totally bottle-fed culture and considered breasts to be only for adult men and not for nursing babies, which is the way some women have come to consider them, then we would regard breast milk differently. Given its possible contamination with toxins, we might even conclude that it was a form of elimination, unsuitable for children. As you can see, there is a degree of cultural value judgment involved in defining the human body and its functions.

Toxic Semen?

The prostate is also a secretory, and, hence, a possibly excretory organ. Prostatic fluid is high in zinc, and it is possible that other metals besides zinc can become attracted to the prostate, such as poisonous cadmium and mercury, since the mechanism whereby the prostate attracts zinc may also operate to attract these less desirable metals. These metals are poisonous because they interfere with normal enzymatic processes, taking the place of the appropriate metal that serves as an integral enzyme component. How this can lead to cancer is not clear, but the poisoning of the prostatic tissue by these metals can be the start. In fact, prostate cancer has been linked to cadmium and mercury poisoning.

Of course, if the prostate is contaminated with cadmium or mercury, it may excrete these metals in the prostatic fluid when the man ejaculates. Semen is typically high in zinc, the normal metal for the prostate. Men with cadmium or mercury poisoned prostates may be eliminating their poisons through orgasms, creating another possible cause of cervical cancer. These metals are known carcinogens.

Other Clothing-Caused Diseases

Of course, like the breast, the prostate is typically constricted by clothing. Some men wear tight underwear, sometimes 24 hours daily, which is known to inhibit sperm production in the testicles by raising the temperature of the organs. Tight belts can interfere with the circulation to the pelvic organs, including the prostate. Clearly, we are altering the environment of the prostate by clothing, and the price we pay for such behavior is usually disease.

If tight clothing can cause cancer, and if eliminatory organs get more cancer because of their handling of carcinogens, it follows that tight clothing around eliminatory organs should cause the most cancer. In fact, the highest incidence of colon cancer occurs in the part of the colon below the belt line. Constriction at the waist, as we explained, inhibits the upward climb of lymphatic fluid from the pelvic organs to the heart. This also applies to the bladder, ovaries, uterus, penis, and testicles, which are all below the belt line. Constriction at the waist can cause problems for all of these organs.

Both these behaviors - wearing constrictive clothing and holding in waste - concentrate toxins in our bodies. Both behaviors are products of our culture. For men and women these behaviors create disease and misery from the cradle onwards. Diverticulitis, kidney stones, cancer. If we live long enough, the misery continues into old age. Men get prostate enlargement with difficulty urinating. And women, they get menopause.

6

Sweating it Out

Menopause is a natural time in a woman's life cycle. It should be no problem, since nature has no investment in suffering. And many women have no problem with menopause, despite their fall in estrogen following the end of their reproductive capacity. Medicine considers menopause a diseased state created by "ovarian failure", which causes reduced estrogen levels and subsequent changes in the woman's body. But if the lowering of estrogen levels causes the problems associated with menopause, why are some women fine despite these hormonal losses?

Menopause has created an industry of products, and books selling those products, to treat menopausal symptoms. None look at the cause of the symptoms, apart from lower estrogen levels. Can we add anything to the barrage of information about this subject? Can menopause have anything to do with elimination?

Sweating to Eliminate

The first clue that this may be the case is discovered when you think about the primary symptoms needing relief – hot flashes, spontaneous sweating, and emotional instability. Why would women sweat during menopause?

We have already discussed the eliminatory function of sweating. Bus drivers who could not urinate or defecate for hours would sweat as an alternative elimination pathway, as we described. When we realize sweating is a form of excretion, and we see menopausal women having hot flashes and sweats, it seems that these women need to eliminate something from their system. Hot flashes are the body's way of heating up to sweat. Why do menopausal women need to sweat?

Hormones and Horses

Medicine tells us that these women sweat because the temperature regulation center in their brains is malfunctioning due to hormonal changes. We are supposed to consider the sweating a symptom of a deranged mind and body, as these menopausal women fall to pieces. It is a fatalistic approach, and the only remedy, say the doctors, is to have these women spend the rest of their lives replacing the hormones lost with new hormones, usually ones that come from the urine of a pregnant female horse. The drug Premarin is such a hormone. The name may reflect that it was *pre*viously *in a mar*e. Millions of pregnant horses are kept confined in dark stalls with catheters inserted into their urethras to extract estrogen from their rich urine and feed it in pill form to menopausal women. It is a multi-billion dollar industry, with 45 million prescriptions written for it in the U.S. alone in 1996, making it an entry in the Guinness Book of World Records. And women taking estrogen are not necessarily helped. Many keep on having hot flashes and sweats. All of them assume a greater chance of developing cancer of the uterus and breasts because of the hormone "therapy".

The source of the confusion is the assumption that menopausal sweating is a symptom of disease, and not simply sweating to eliminate toxins. Why would menopausal women need to eliminate more toxins during menopause than before menopause, leading to these sweats? It is because while menstruating, toxins had been regularly removed via the menstrual flow. Having stopped this form of elimination with the onset of menopause, toxins that had been eliminated in the menstrual flow must find new outlets for release from the body. The colon, kidneys, and lungs can take some of the slack. But sweating is also a needed outlet.

Antiperspirants

Making matters worse, many women wear antiperspirant, inhibiting their sweat response. If the body needs to sweat under the pressure of this added toxin load, but cannot because of antiperspirants, then the toxin levels begin to increase in the body. This can lead to toxemia and the feelings of irritability and other nervous system abnormalities associated with menopause. Ultimately, the body can stand its toxin level no longer. In the middle of the day or night, without notice, the woman feels a hot flash as her body decides it's time to sweat out the toxins. The woman finally breaks a sweat and excretes some of the toxins. These spontaneous sweats of menopause, then, are the body's way of forcing perspiration to occur in order to eliminate.

Testing Our Menopause Theory

We tested this theory about menopausal sweating by asking ten menopausal women to take daily steam baths or saunas to sweat. We reasoned that if we were correct about the cause of menopausal sweating, then we might be able to eliminate the need for spontaneous sweating by having the women take a deliberate, controlled sweat. This would eliminate the toxins and make spontaneous sweating unnecessary. We received passes for the women to the local YWCA which had a sauna and steam room, and asked the women to sweat daily for two months to see the effect.

Four of the ten women didn't follow through. Their schedules did not allow them to commit to daily sweats. Actually, these women expressed disdain for sweating at all. Many women abhor the feeling of being hot and sweaty. It's part of their cultural conditioning. So these women dropped out of the study, and their hot flashes and sweats continued.

Of the remaining six women, one could not sweat easily, and felt overheated trying to do so. She continued to have hot flashes. As for the remaining five, they stopped having hot flashes and spontaneous sweats. Most felt relief by the end of the second week. Each of these five women had been on various treatments for menopause, none of which had worked. Sweating it out was all that helped.

Nature or Nurture?

Menopausal discomfort is a cultural disease. When we went to Fiji to perform research on breast disease, which we discuss in our book, ***Get It Off!***, we also took the opportunity to ask Fijian women in traditional villages about their experience of menopause. "What's that?" they asked. "You know," we explained. "When you get older and stop being able to have children. Is that a difficult time for Fijian women?"

The women looked at us with confusion. They don't have a problem with that time of life, they explained. When they stop having periods they go to the doctor, wondering if they are pregnant. When they are told that it is just their time to stop having babies, they heave a sigh of relief, and that's all. They don't even have a word for that time in life. Menopause has no Fijian equivalent. We observed that these women do not use antiperspirants, either, and they sweat comfortably. In other words, their culture is not sweat-phobic, like western cultures.

Strange Cultural Practices

We did learn something else interesting in Fiji. While Fijian culture is liberal about sweating, it does have some strange hygiene behaviors that create health problems. Since we are medical anthropologists, we find it more interesting living with the people of the cultures we visit, rather than staying in a westernized resort. Because of the poverty there, many Fijians have poor sanitation facilities. I remember the first time I needed to go defecate. It was our first exposure to these conditions and to this culture, and we were staying with a family in their shack. When I asked where the bathroom was, the host pointed to an outhouse a hundred yards away. I went to the outhouse with relative urgency, only to discover that there was no toilet paper. Returning to the host for instructions, I asked, "Where is the toilet paper?" I was promptly handed a bucket. "What is this for?" The reply was a brief glance at the stream passing nearby.

Wipe or Wash?

This was the first time we were forced to wash our bottoms with water. By one week, our anuses felt healthier than ever before.

When you think about it, if you had poop on your arm, would you rub it off with dry paper, or wash it off with water? Of course, you'd use water. Yet, U.S. culture almost exclusively promotes toilet tissue. Europeans, as well as some other cultures throughout the world, have been using water and bidets for quite some time. But the paper industry must be extremely powerful in the U.S.. Besides, discomfort with excretions makes it unlikely that Americans would readily touch their stool with their hands while cleaning their bottoms. Putting toilet paper between the hand and the poop provides the culturally required distance.

Toilet Paper

The family with the water bucket was an Indian family in Fiji. East Indians constitute about half of the Fijian population. When we later stayed with a black Fijian family, we discovered another interesting hygiene behavior. In the outhouse were strips of newspaper. It was clear that these were not to be read, but were for some other function. We soon realized their purpose. Too poor to buy toilet tissue, and desirous of copying western ways, these Fijians were using the *Fiji Times* to clean themselves. Don't use the newspaper coupons to buy toilet paper. Use the coupons *as* toilet paper!

This would be more amusing if it wasn't for the fact that

newspaper is filled with toxic chemicals, from dioxins that cause cancer, to inks, glues, and other chemical products, none of which you would want on your moist anus. Not surprisingly, rectal cancer is high in Fiji.

So is cervical cancer. And the cause is the same. After urinating women dab themselves dry with the Sunday comics. And menstruating women use wads of newspaper as an absorbent while having their periods.

The experience of washing with water, followed by our discovery of this novel use of the *Fiji Times*, led us to research the safety of toilet tissue used in the U.S. Indeed, numerous articles describe skin disease in the anal region caused by toilet tissue. It follows from the nature of toilet tissue. This product is designed to fall apart in the water so it does not clog the sewer lines. It is held together by glue that dissolves in water. This means that it will partially dissolve on the anus and vagina as soon as it touches moisture, applying glue and other chemical products to the body. Repeated daily application of this paper to the body leads to dermatitis, anal itching, allergic reactions, and increases the toxin load of the tissues.

Different Strokes for Different Folks

For the Fijians we met it was a surprise to learn that newspaper is a poor toilet tissue and sanitary pad. Their culture had conditioned them to its use. We seemed almost ridiculous in our concerns about it. Like the members of all cultures, they resisted changing their ways.

We are all victims of our culture and its ways. We are beneficiaries of some of its ways, as well. But the price we must pay for the benefits is frequently our health. However, there is something we can do about it.

7

Putting the Pieces Together

Let us summarize the information we have given you in the preceding chapters.

- When you have to defecate or fart and hold it in, you create extra pressure in your colon. Doing this time and again may cause pockets to form in the colon wall, called diverticula. These pockets can get infected, causing diverticulitis.

- How do you prevent diverticulitis? Defecate when you need to and don't hold back gas when it wants to leave.

- When you need to urinate and hold it in, you create extra pressure in the bladder and kidneys. This causes the bladder to press against the prostate gland, which, if done time and again, may lead to prostate enlargement. The urine will concentrate, increasing its likelihood of forming salt crystals and other deposits, which, if done time and again, may lead to stone formation. And the bladder distended with concentrated urine may become irritated, increasing its likelihood of developing infections.

- How do you prevent prostate enlargement, kidney stones, and bladder infections? Urinate when you need to.

- If you are a menstruating woman, tampon use can irritate the vagina and cervix and may chemically contaminate the

51

tissue. If done time and again, then this may lead to mucus discharge, abnormal cell growth, and possibly cancer.

◆ How do you prevent cervical dysplasia and cervical cancer? Don't use tampons.

◆ Toxins that are being eliminated with the menstrual flow may irritate the uterus, causing cramping.

◆ How do you prevent menstrual cramping? Don't use antiperspirants or wear tight clothing, drink more, urinate more, and sweat more.

◆ If you are a menopausal woman and experience hot flashes, sweats, and mood swings, it is a sign that toxins are accumulating in your body due to a cessation of menstruation as an elimination process.

◆ To avoid menopausal discomforts avoid antiperspirants, drink more, urinate more, and sweat more.

In each case it is the same story. When your body is telling you it needs to eliminate, whether it be urine, stool, sweat, or blood, let it. It is an amazingly simple and obvious realization. When we need to eliminate, we should let ourselves do so. Yet, few of us consistently heed that message.

We all have held in gas, even to the extent of a great deal of cramping pain, when letting it go would be socially unthinkable. We all have felt the urge to defecate, but held it in because a restroom was not handy, or because a restroom was handy but it was a public restroom and we didn't want to use it for whatever reason, or because we just didn't want to take the time at that moment to stop and poop.

We all have felt the need to urinate, but held it in because we were on the freeway and we just couldn't stop, or because we were walking in a part of the city with no restaurants or alleys or bushes, or because we just didn't want to take the time to find a place to pee and we knew we could hold it in a bit longer.

We all have felt the need to stay dry for some social occasion and tried applying some substances to our armpits to prevent embarrassing wet circles on our clothes and body odor.

We are all guilty of the sin of self-oppression. Actually, it is our social selves that oppress our natural selves. We have all learned the cultural art of self-control. We have become domesticated.

Must this conflict exist between our nature and our civility? Can we express the beast while maintaining our bearing?

There are some things we can do to ensure that we get our personal needs met.

- Time your activities to allow for bathroom breaks.

- Anticipate needing a restroom and make sure one will be available when needed.

- Expect the need to eliminate after eating and drinking, which stimulate the digestion and kidneys.

- Make sure that your children eliminate when needed. Tell them how important it is to go when they have to, and that holding it in can cause disease. Remind them to urinate before they go to bed.

- If it makes you more comfortable, travel with toilet seat covers and other personal items that you might need in a restroom, such as soap, a towel, and a plastic water bottle for washing.

- When you are in a public restroom, observe strict cleanliness habits. Realize that the most handled areas in the room are the flusher handles, the sink handles, and the door handles. People with infectious diseases of the digestive tract, genital tract, or urinary system will touch those handles. It may be best to touch all handles with a paper towel in hand.

This last point is one reason why many people resist going to public restrooms, making them hold it in instead. Public restrooms can sometimes be very unpleasant places. And you never know for sure what may be happening behind closed stall doors. Of course, there are plush restrooms in fancy hotels, where you get an attendant to handle the handles for you. These luxurious chambers are our culture's finest attempt to bring good taste to toileting. If only we could hire others to do the entire business.

There is a business that cares very much about your waste. It's the healthcare business. You can tell a great deal about the general health of the body by the waste it puts out. The smell, color, and consistency of stool and urine are still regarded as important diagnostic information, as they have been for millennia. It was by tasting urine that ancient physicians discovered the key symptom of diabetes that is still considered its key feature by modern medicine. The urine of these patients tastes sweet. Today we know it is from excreting sugar in the urine. The name "diabetes mellitus", in fact, means "sweet urine". These days, of course, they use machines to do the "tasting".

So have a look before you flush. Here is what to look for.

The Scoop on Poop

The diet is the most important factor that determines stool color. In addition, as we mentioned, the usual brown color is from two pigments produced by the liver as breakdown products of hemoglobin, which is the pigment of red blood cells.

If the stool is brown, you have an average, well-balanced diet.

If it is light brown, you are on a milk diet.

If it is brownish-black, you are on a high meat diet.

Yellow signifies you ate rhubarb and/or lots of fat.

Green may mean you ate spinach.

Black stool is created by bleeding in the stomach or intestines, or by bismuth (as in the product Pepto-Bismol), or by iron salts.

Grayish-white or clay-colored stool suggests liver or gallbladder obstruction, preventing the bile from entering the intestine.

Red stool suggests bleeding in the rectum or colon, or may simply mean that you ate beets or lots of tomatoes.

The unpleasant smell of feces is due to methane, hydrogen sulfide, and methyl mercaptan, which are gaseous bacterial products. Meat diets produce a strong odor, while milk and vegetable diets produce a milder smell. A very foul odor indicates alkaline feces; acidic feces smell sour or rancid.

Antibiotics kill intestinal bacteria, and this alters the appearance and smell of feces. The stool may become bulky, contain more undigested material, often have a greenish-gray color, and may be odorless. There may be a marked increase in mucus, which is a sign of irritation. Diarrhea with watery stools may occur.

There is more to tell from feces if you have a microscope and wish to look for signs of parasites. Medical labs can perform tests to tell the fat, starch, and other components of stool samples. But for a general snapshot of how your digestion is doing, the color and smell tells a great deal.

When Urine Formed

You can tell some things about your health from the color and smell of your urine, as well.

Normally, urine is pale yellow and quite clear. If it is colorless, it indicates dilution, and suggests that you have had too much water relative to salt, and that you need to eliminate water. Dark yellow indicates concentration, and suggests that you need more water and should urinate more frequently.

Milky urine suggests pus and infection in the urinary tract. Or it could simply mean that you had a high fat meal and are urinating out fat.

Orange urine is associated with hemoglobin breakdown, foods, or drugs.

Red urine can result from eating beets, or can result from bleeding.

Greenish urine suggests liver disease. Dirty-blue or green

urine is seen when urine is putrefying, as well as in typhus and cholera.

Brown-red and dark-brown urine can reflect high concentration or disease associated with fever.

Bright red, reddish-brown, brown-black, or black urine suggests blood and disease.

The odor of urine is considered only when it is fresh. Volatile fatty acids give urine its normal smell. Bacteria degrading urea to ammonia gives it an ammonia smell. A fruity smell of acetone appears in a metabolic condition called ketosis, which may accompany dieting and fasting. Asparagus can give urine a characteristic odor, too.

You should get to know the normal color and smell of your waste products so you can tell when something changes. A change in color can reflect a change in diet. But it can also be a sign of a health problem that needs attention.

While we have been focusing on only these two forms of elimination, the same self-awareness should apply to all excretions from your body. Mucus suggests irritation. Red and brown suggest blood. These simple visual indications can be your first sign of a problem. If something seems abnormal, get it checked out. Ask yourself what you have been doing, including what you have been eating, that may have created the abnormality.

Soma's son, Troy, was once sent home from school in a panic due to apparent blood in his urine. The school nurse suspected kidney damage, and expected Troy would need to be rushed to the hospital. Soma reflected before reacting, and remembered that she had served beets the night before, which Troy relished. The nurse never actually checked his urine for blood. The urine cleared up in a day, but Troy now has anxiety whenever he eats beets.

The moral of the story is to think before you panic. Most of what you are eliminating is a product of what you have taken into your body. So don't be afraid when you see red. Be thoughtful. And discover its cause.

Drug Side Effects

We have discussed the need to answer the call of nature when it comes. When the cause of waste retention is our culturally trained ability to wait, it is a simple issue of changing your attitudes and behaviors. However, for many people, constipation and gas are an endless nightmare. They would love to sit on the toilet and let it all out. The same thing goes for people needing to empty their bladder. We have assumed that the cause of the retention is our cultural attitudes and behaviors. Sometimes, however, the cause is in the drugs doctors prescribe.

Bladder and intestinal function are regulated by intricate hormonal and neural mechanisms involving the brain, liver, kidneys, and more. When drugs are used to treat a condition, they alter the body's physiology and chemistry. Frequently, this alteration affects unintended parts of the body, altering their function, as well. These unintended effects of a drug are called side effects. They accompany all drug usage. As a result, a person can be given a drug for Parkinson's Disease, for example, and it can cause a reduction in intestinal activity as a side effect, as well as causing urinary retention. To stop the tremors of Parkinson's, the drug interferes with a central biochemical mechanism that also is involved in allowing the intestines and bladder to contract. The result is constipation and difficulty urinating.

There are many drugs that cause constipation and urinary difficulty as a side effect. Some drugs create diarrhea and excessive urination as their side effect. Some drugs can make you sweat profusely, while others make you unable to sweat at all. Some drugs give you gas. So it is important to consider the drugs you are taking as a potential source of interference with your waste disposal system.

Life's a Gas

We must make one further point about intestinal gas. We have urged the reader to allow the fumes of digestion to readily pass to the outside, whether in the form of burps or farts. However, we must also be sensitive to the cultural reality that limits some forms of personal expression. How can we maintain our civility without losing our health by holding in gas?

Here are some common sense guidelines for farting:

- Try to fart down wind from others.

- When you fart, don't make an issue of it. It's not like a sneeze. You don't have to say excuse me, or hold your hand over your bottom. If you don't make an issue out of it, no mature person will.

- When an immature person does make an issue out of it, so what? Their turn will come.

- Never say your farts don't smell. To others, they do.

- Try to marry someone with a bad sense of smell.

- Check your diet to figure out what is giving you extra gas and stop eating those foods. You may have to experiment by eliminating one food at a time and then adding it back to see its effect. You may be surprised to discover that the cabbage, ice cream, and onions you love give you gas.

- Defecating can sometimes eliminate farts.

- Be kind to others who fart. What goes around, comes around.

Knowing the Cause is the Key to Health

If you have a health problem, discovering its cause is the most important thing you can do to begin healing. Without knowing the cause, you cannot properly treat a condition. Until the cause is removed, all treatment will be temporary. This serves the economic interests of a treatment industry. But it does not serve your health interests.

Your health is up to you. You are a human animal, living in

a modern, westernized culture. You must find ways to live within that culture and still satisfy your natural needs to eliminate waste. When nature calls, it's up to you to answer. If you don't answer, nature leaves a message — in the form of pain and discomfort. If you still ignore the call, it will leave more forceful messages, such as disease. And if you still refuse the call, nature may hang up and disconnect your line.

Nature calls you through your senses. Your pains and pleasures are nature's messages that serve as your lifestyle guideposts. We can play the cultural game, so long as we observe the natural signs. Otherwise, we get penalized.

SELF STUDIES

Connecting with your senses, then, is your way to connect with health. That is why we have developed SELF STUDIES. These are your way to see for yourself, on yourself, how certain lifestyle changes can improve your health.

We came upon the idea of SELF STUDIES as a result of our bra and breast cancer work. We began to receive reports from women with fibrocystic breast disease that their breasts felt better after no longer wearing bras. We then suggested that other women try testing this for themselves, and they felt major changes within weeks, if not days. As our research efforts turned to migraines and head elevation, we suggested that people try that simply lifestyle change to see if they had been sleeping too flat. And they, too, felt a difference within weeks, if not days.

To encourage people to participate in SELF STUDIES we have started the Self Study Center. It can be found on the Internet at www.selfstudycenter.org. This free service describes what we believe are the cultural causes of various diseases, and suggests risk-free, cost-free lifestyle changes that people can try for themselves. The taboo topics we have covered in this book are on the site, as well.

We hope that the information we are giving allows people to adopt healthful lifestyles. Living healthfully is the way to prevent disease. And eliminating unhealthy lifestyles is the way to recover from disease.

When people are suffering from disease, they typically ask what they need to do to get better. Actually, they should be asking what they should stop doing that has been making them sick in the first place.

Sometimes we need to take something to get better. But sometimes we just need to eliminate.

The Three New Laws of Nature

Through our work as medical anthropologists, we have discovered three new laws of nature that humans must obey for health.

- ◆ Elevate the top half of your bed 30-degrees while sleeping, and sleep on your back. (See **Get It Up!**)

- ◆ Wear lose clothes that allow proper blood and lymphatic circulation. (See **Get It Off!**)

- ◆ Listen to the calls of nature. When you have to go, go!

Nature will not argue about these issues, despite what the culture says. These truths are self-evident to those who perform SELF STUDIES. Your body will let you know what makes it feel healthy or ill.

If you have broken these natural laws of human health, and you now suffer from disease, it is never too late to change your lifestyle. As soon as you end the insults to your body it can begin to heal. So long as you are alive you are capable of healing. Keep your courage. Place your faith in the powers of life that have animated your body and have maintained its integrity since your conception. Honor that power in yourself. Honor yourself as the possessor of that power. It is the only power you really need.

It takes maturity, desire, and self-reflection to be healthy. Sometimes, it may make you go against the fashions of the times. But your health is worth it.

The choice is yours.

8

Answers To Embarrassing Questions

Let's say that you agree with all we have said thus far. You firmly resolve to eliminate when nature first suggests, rather than to wait for nature to demand. You agree to lower your resistance to addressing eliminatory issues in your life, and resolve to improve the health of your colon, bladder, kidneys, uterus or prostate, and the rest of your body that relies so greatly on your allowing waste to issue forth from your eliminatory system when necessary.

But what if it's inconvenient?

Is this book too idealistic to suggest that we can accommodate our natural needs while remaining civilized?

Before you say, "Yes!" let us present some challenging social situations and discuss ways of managing them for optimal health and civility. To make the issues seem more tangible we will present them in fictionalized "letter to the expert" form, like you would see in a newspaper column such as "Dear Miss Manners", or, perhaps in this case, "Dear Miss Ill-Manners".

Letter #1

Dear Syd and Soma,

I was traveling all day and was running late when I finally arrived at Houston for an important business meeting. The flight I had been on circled the airport for 30 minutes before it finally landed. By the time we hit the runway my bladder felt like it was about to burst. As the plane jerked to a dead stop the seatbelt dug into my belly so hard that I think I lost a drop or two in my underwear. I began to perspire as I waited for the seatbelt sign to be extinguished. I almost couldn't stand up to leave my seat because of the pain in my bladder.

Naturally, I was at the back of the plane, so it took another 10 minutes to inch my way up the aisle. By the time I got inside the terminal I was sweating profusely. I headed for the nearest bathroom, which was about 100 yards down the terminal hallway. As I propelled my aching body forward, my only thoughts were of bladder relief. Anticipation heightened my sense of need, and my bladder began to contract involuntarily. I was a desperate man. It felt not one moment too soon when I finally managed to swim my way against a tide of new arrivals to get to the mens' restroom. You can imagine my utter horror when I saw the "Restroom Closed for Repairs" sign.

For a moment I just stood there. I was no longer an executive from Des Moines. Now I was a desperate animal longing for primal satisfaction of my urinary needs. I peeked around the wall to see if the restroom was usable. The lights were out and the plumbing was dismantled. Across the hallway of the terminal was the ladies' restroom. I contemplated my choices. The nearest restroom was too far away for me to possibly reach without losing bladder control. I couldn't just urinate in the hallway. And all the stalls in the ladies' restroom have doors. One could be discrete. It's an emergency.

As I was about to enter the ladies' restroom a woman pulling a yellow wash bucket emerged. I paused and felt such guilt and shame that it was the last straw for my poor bladder. A puddle formed around my new wing-tipped shoes. I hoped the woman with the bucket wouldn't notice, but it's her job to notice such things.

"The men's restroom is out of order," she said with a straight face. "But please don't do that out here."

I now have nightmares about public restrooms and make sure that I never drink while traveling so I don't need to urinate until safely in my hotel room or back at home. Of course, since my last kidney stone my doctor told me to drink more. But who can drink when you can't pee? They go together.

Can you advise me of what to do if the above situation ever happens again?

Signed,
Wet in Houston

Dear Wet,

The next time, pee while still on the plane. If you can't until they land, then go in the plane once they do land. If you had to vomit you would. They have airsickness bags for vomiting passengers. The need to urgently urinate is no less honorable than the need to vomit, and is a lot neater. Assert your bladder rights! And if you have to crash a ladies' restroom in an emergency, just yell, "Tally Ho! An emergency ladies! A man must enter. Please forgive!" Give a moment for a scream and if you hear none, enter. But keep your eyes down, go directly to the stall, close the door, do your business, and then quickly leave, without looking back.

Letter #2

Dear Syd and Soma,

My husband has a fart problem. I don't know how he managed to hold them in when we were dating. But when we got married, forget it. He's proud of some of them. I could be in the middle of making dinner or doing the dishes and he'll come over to me with this big grin on his face, turn his back to me, and whistle a happy tune. I've always appreciated music, but this is taking it too far.

The other night, though, I had a fright, which is why I'm writing you. We were in bed and since it was cold that night we had an extra blanket on the bed, you know, to make it cozy and snugly. Wouldn't you know it but old windbag got started, if you know what I mean, and there was that toot and smell again. He's always complaining of gas pains, and he felt such relief on getting that one out that he started feeling amorous.

Well, I'm mortified to tell anyone this, but as we were making love, he leaned on my belly and I let out a silent, but especially pungent flatus. It took no time for Buster (that's not his real name) to become aware of my deed. Needless to say, I felt ashamed and soiled by the experience. I haven't wanted to have sex again since then. What should I do? Are farts contagious?

Signed,
Windy

Dear Windy,

Birds do it. We don't think bees do it. Educated fleas probably do it. Humans certainly do it. Flatus is natural. Don't fight it. If you hold it in, it could give you disease.

Farts are not contagious, although if they are

associated with bacteria, the bacteria could theoretically be transferred from one person to another through intimate contact, possibly spreading the farts. Most flatus, however, consists of benign farts, which reflect personal digestive function. These farts are safe to be around, although the environment may become disagreeably odiferous.

As for your new sexual problem, it seems that you have been embarrassed by the most insignificant of human realities. If your man loves you, he does so for your human qualities. This is one of them. Besides, it's your turn now.

Letter #3

Dear Syd and Soma,

One week out of every month I feel like Hell. My breasts get sore, I get a migraine that lasts days, my uterus cramps like a knife is in me, I get pimples, I feel like I want to die, and my boyfriend says I get bitchy because I'm not interested in sex at those times. Sometimes I feel like punching him in the nuts. My doctor, a man, told me my monthly problems are normal and I should get used to them. He can give me drugs if it really gets bad, which it does. But I hate using drugs. What can I do?

Signed,
Not Really a Bitch

Dear Not Really,

*For your migraines, you need to sleep with the top half of your body elevated. Your head is getting too much pressure and congestion from lying too flat. See our book, **Get It Up! Revealing the Simple Surprising Lifestyle that Causes Migraines, Alzheimer's, Stroke, Glaucoma, Sleep Apnea, Impotence,...and More!***

*As for your breast soreness, you need to get rid of your bra. Bras are tight and can constrict the breasts, impairing the circulation. When you are about to have a period, your breasts are larger from a general body swelling that happens at that time of the month due to elevated estrogen levels. If you are wearing the same sized bra all month, larger breasts make the bra even tighter, leading to extra constriction, pain, fluid build-up, and cyst formation. See our book, **Get It Off! Understanding the Cause of Breast Pain, Cysts, and Cancer, Illustrated with a***

Little Breast Play.

As for your pimples and cramps, these can be caused by toxins that your body is trying to eliminate. Try taking a steam bath or sauna or a hot bath to get hot enough to sweat, and sweat for about 10 minutes each day. Make sure you replace salts as well as water following sweating. Try mineral water with salty food, or some commercial beverages sold for fluid replacement.

As for your boyfriend, it is hard to have sympathy for his lack of empathy. If he gets out of hand and tries to insist that you satisfy his growing needs, you may want to get him under the covers and then fart. We'll send you a letter from a reader named Windy that may be helpful.

Letter #4

Dear Syd and Soma,

I have read all your books and think you make real sense. Unfortunately, your books weren't around for the first 65 years of my life, and now I'm a mess.

I was an insurance agency manager. I retired two years ago. While in some ways I wish I were still conducting those Monday morning meetings, I must admit that I'm relieved. Over the years my diverticulitis would get so bad that I could hardly sit still. There were times I had to fabricate a lie to get away to pass gas, saying I had a call to make and closing my office door. I'll never forget my embarrassment when my new secretary walked into my office one foggy day when my foghorn was blowing rather uncontrollably. She tried to hide it, but I could see her discomfort. I think she tried holding her breath.

I found that I was in the restroom so much I thought I'd have phones installed in the stalls. An uncomfortable situation once happened when two of my agents came into the restroom while I was sitting and reading the *Wall Street Journal*. I had a bad case of diarrhea that day, and the smell must have been horrific. The agents reflexively gasped and one said, "Wow! It smells like someone died in here!" The other laughed. And then there was a moment of silence and a whisper. I think one of them looked under the stall door and recognized my shoes. They did their business in silence and left. Somehow, I think I lost their respect. Our relationship never felt the same since.

When my prostate began to bother me I spent even more time at the restroom. It's ironic that for my entire career I hardly ever went to the restroom when at work. By the end of my career, I couldn't get out of the restroom.

Now that I'm retired I no longer have Monday morning meetings at the office. I have Monday morning doctor appointments. My urologist, Dr. Stone, wants to drill open my prostate, inserting the drill up my penis. I told him I'd think about it. Do you think this doctor's parents know what he does to people for a living?

My proctologist, Dr. Butts, wants to operate on my diverticulitis, and says I may need to have a section of my colon removed. There is the possibility that my colon will have to exit my side. I don't feel bad enough to believe that such drastic measures will be needed. But my doctor has warned me that my condition can lead to infection and death. He says I'll need surgery sooner or later, and it might as well be sooner. He can do it by inserting surgical tools up my anus and rectum.

If they turn me on the side, could both work on me at the same time?

Is there any alternative to having these doctors probe my private parts?

Signed,
An Old Fart

Dear Old Fart,

As long as your body is alive and has the desire to live, it has the ability to heal. That is, provided that you remove the cause of the problem. While it is true that in old age we reap what we have sown in youth, there is still time to right a wrong.

Make sure you urinate as fully and as often as possible. You have created a vicious cycle of trouble by holding in urine. The overfilled bladder compressed the prostate. This caused the prostate to enlarge to resist the compression. This, in turn, limited the outflow of urine from your bladder, preventing complete emptying and making the bladder fuller. The cycle then continues.

Once you stop holding in urine, the cause of the prostate enlargement ends. If you now have the luxury of eliminating at will, you may be able to keep your bladder empty, and keep your prostate from getting any larger. The prostate may or may not get smaller under lower pressure from the bladder. But it should get no larger. If you shun surgery, you may not need it so long as you can urinate. If you are open to the surgery but don't feel completely desperate, consider the possible side effects related to having someone drill a hole through your prostate and into your bladder. Once the normal bleeding stops and your penis recovers so you no longer feel burning and pain while urinating, and assuming that you do not get a bladder infection or lose your ability to hold in urine by having your bladder sphincter damaged, will you be better off, or worse off?

The same argument applies to diverticulitis. When you allow yourself to defecate when needed and pass gas when needed, the cause of your diverticulitis will be removed, and the body can start healing. As with the prostate, however, do not expect that the outcome of years of self-abuse will vanish within weeks or months. It took you years to get this way. Healing will take years, as well. But keep in mind that healing is a process. So long as you are healing, you are moving in the right direction. As for surgical intervention, again, this is up to you. But don't automatically assume that you will be better off for the surgery. Surgery, unlike these diseases, is irreversible.

Of course, there may be situations where surgery can save a life. The surgeons will point out these examples to sell their services. But what about the situations that would have resolved better without surgery? Consumer beware! Surgery should be a last resort. It's something you have when your body cannot heal itself. At those times you have nothing to lose. If you still have something to lose, you must decide whether to put your faith in medicine, or in yourself.

As an insurance agency manager, at least you probably have the right kind of insurance. Insurance makes it easier to put your faith in medicine. Nobody pays you for putting your faith in yourself. Typically, your only payment is good health.

Some Interesting References

Wynne-Jones G.
Flatus retention is the major factor in diverticular disease.
Lancet. 1975 Aug 2;2(7927):211-2.

Ornstein MH, Littlewood ER, Baird IM, Fowler J, North WR, Cox AG.
Are fibre supplements really necessary in diverticular disease of the colon? A controlled clinical trial.
Br Med J (Clin Res Ed). 1981 Apr 25;282(6273):1353-6.

Nickel JC, Downey J, Feliciano AE Jr, Hennenfent B.
Repetitive prostatic massage therapy for chronic refractory prostatitis: the Philippine experience.
Tech Urol. 1999 Sep;5(3):146-51.

Evans JM, Owens TP Jr, Zerbe DM, Rohren CH.
Venous obstruction due to a distended urinary bladder.
Mayo Clin Proc. 1995 Nov;70(11):1077-9.

Schild SE, Casale HE, Bellefontaine LP.
Movements of the prostate due to rectal and bladder distension: implications for radiotherapy.
Med Dosim. 1993 Spring;18(1):13-5.

Kopesky K, Schwartz R, Silver D.
Lower extremity edema from bladder compression of the iliac veins.
J Vasc Surg. 1988 Jun;7(6):778-80.

Guin JD.
Contact dermatitis to perfume in paper products.
J Am Acad Dermatol. 1981 Jun;4(6):733-4.

Keith L, Reich W, Bush IM.
Toilet paper dermatitis.
JAMA. 1969 Jul 14;209(2):269.

Mauss J.
[Anal hygiene using water spray].
ZFA (Stuttgart). 1980 Apr 30;56(12):881-3. German.

Banov L Jr.
Anal hygiene; its prophylactic value.
J S C Med Assoc. 1966 Sep;62(9):357-9.

Walker K.
[Report on anal hygiene].
Landarzt. 1967 Sep 30;43(27):1321-5. German.

Blecher P, Korting HC.
Tolerance to different toilet paper preparations: toxicological and allergological aspects.
Dermatology. 1995;191(4):299-304.

Piletta-Zanin PA, Pasche-Koo F, Auderset PC, Huggengerger D, Saurat JH, Hauser C.
Detection of formaldehyde in moistened baby toilet tissues.
Contact Dermatitis. 1998 Jan;38(1):46.

de Groot AC.
Vesicular dermatitis of the hands secondary to perianal allergic contact dermatitis caused by preservatives in moistened toilet tissues.
Contact Dermatitis. 1997 Mar;36(3):173-4.

Guimaraens D, Conde-Salazar L, Gonzalez MA.
Allergic contact dermatitis on the hands from chloromethylisothiazolinone in moist toilet paper.
Contact Dermatitis. 1996 Oct;35(4):254.

Hulsmans RF, van der Kley AM, Weyland JW, de Groot AC.
[Replacement of Kathon CG by Euxyl K 400 in cosmetics; from the frying pan into the fire]?
Ned Tijdschr Geneeskd. 1992 Mar 21;136(12):587-9. Dutch.

de Groot AC, Baar TJ, Terpstra H, Weyland JW.
Contact allergy to moist toilet paper.
Contact Dermatitis. 1991 Feb;24(2):135-6.

Friedrich EG Jr.
Tampon effects on vaginal health.
Clin Obstet Gynecol. 1981 Jun;24(2):395-406.

Danielson RW.
Vaginal ulcers caused by tampons.
Am J Obstet Gynecol. 1983 Jul 1;146(5):547-9.

Roberts TM.
Vaginal health effects of tampon use: implications for vaginitis.
Nurse Pract. 1994 Sep;19(9):75-6.

Oram C, Beck J.
The tampon: investigated and challenged.
Women Health. 1981 Fall-Winter;6(3-4):105-22.

Maguire DL Jr.
Tampon vaginitis.
J S C Med Assoc. 1966 Nov;62(11):432-3.

Khanolkar VR., Suryabai B.
Cancer in relation to usages: three new types in India.
[A cancer of the lower trunk and groin associated with the
Deccani Hindu custom of wearing –even while bathing – a tight-
fitting form of trousers known as a *dhoti*.]
Archives of Path. 1945 40:351-361

Adatto K, Doebele KG, Galland L, Granowetter L.
Behavioral factors and urinary tract infection.
JAMA. 1979 Jun 8;241(23):2525-6.

Postscript

The issues we have raised in this book pertain to the eliminatory needs of the human animal. We wish to point out that these same natural needs are shared by other animals with whom humans live, such as dogs and cats. Many loving dog owners unknowingly cause their animal companions great pain and suffering by keeping the creatures indoors and unable to eliminate. While cats can use a litter box, they may refrain from using it if the litter material is offensive from overuse or from an obnoxious (to the cat) litter material. When pets hold in their waste they can develop constipation and other digestive troubles, as well as kidney and bladder disease. Please consider the eliminatory needs of your pet. If you don't want them getting sick, or getting the house messy, then let them "get it out" outside.

ABOUT THE AUTHORS

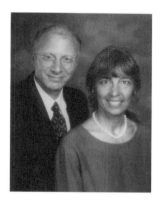

Sydney Ross Singer and **Soma Grismaijer** are a husband-and-wife research team dedicated to uncovering the lifestyle causes of disease. Medical anthropologists and co-authors of, *Dressed To Kill: The Link Between Breast Cancer and Bras* (Avery, 1995), *Get It Up!, Get It Off!,* and *Get It Out!,* (ISCD Press, 2000-2001) this dynamic duo is known worldwide for their willingness to stand up to the profit-oriented, treatment focused medical system.

Sydney Ross Singer received a B.S. in biology from the University of Utah in 1979. He then spent two years in the biochemistry Ph.D. program at Duke University, followed by another two years at Duke in the anthropology Ph.D. program, receiving a Master's Degree. He then attended the University of Texas Medical Branch (UTMB) at Galveston, Texas on a full academic scholarship, where he spent one year in the medical humanities Ph.D. program, and received an additional two years training in medical school.

Soma Grismaijer received an associate's degree from the College of Marin in the behavioral sciences, and a bachelor of arts from Sonoma State University in environmental studies and planning. In addition, she is an American Board of Opticianry-certified optician. She has been the President and Executive Director of the Good Shepherd Foundation since 1980, a charitable organization dedicated to the elimination of human and animal suffering.

Together, Singer and Grismaijer started the Institute for the Study of Culturogenic Disease in 1991. Their first project was the M.D. (Medical Demystification) Crusade, informing the public of the hazards of medicine and how to prevent them. The Crusade included the Medication Side Effects Hotline, and a national lecture tour explaining the nature of doctors, medicine, and health. Following their research into the cause of breast cancer and the publication of **Dressed To Kill**, Singer and Grismaijer traveled around the world bringing their health message to millions of people. Currently, they are spearheading an international campaign to educate people about various culturogenic diseases, explaining how to prevent and cure a host of conditions considered a "mystery" by modern medicine . In addition, they have begun an Internet based SELF STUDY CENTER, at selfstudycenter.org, to help people practice health self-care by trying certain lifestyle changes.

Singer and Grismaijer, and their 9 year-old Solomon, practice what they preach in Hawaii, on a 67-acre tropical rainforest preserve.

<u>*Welcome to the Medical Revolution!*</u>

ISCD Press Books
by
SINGER and *GRISMAIJER*

This is original information with new medical insights and discoveries that are only found at **ISCD Press!**

Get It Up! **Revealing the Simple Surprising Lifestyle that Causes Migraines, Alzheimer's, Stroke, Glaucoma, Sleep Apnea, Impotence, ...and More!**
ISBN 1-930858-00-0

Get It Off! **Understanding the Cause of Breast Pain, Cysts, and Cancer, Illustrated with A Little Breast Play.** ISBN 1-930858-01-9

Get It Out! **Eliminating the Cause of Diverticulitis, Kidney Stones, Bladder Infections, Cervical Dysplasia, PMS, Menopausal Discomfort, Prostate Enlargement, ...and More!**
ISBN 1-930858-02-7

The Doctor Is Out! **Exposing the High Blood Pressure, Low Thyroid and Diabetes Scams.**
ISBN 1-930858-04-3

Available at **www.ISCDPress.com**

ISCD Press, P.O. Box 1880, Pahoa, HI 96778 USA
(808) 935-5563   email: iscd@ISCDPress.com